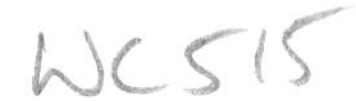

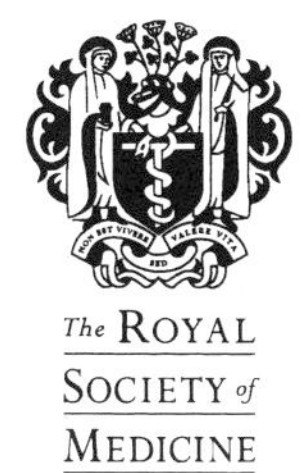

Influenza: human and avian in Practice

ND EDITION

Roy Jennings
Emeritus Professor, Section of Infection and Immunity, Division of Genomic Medicine, University of Sheffield, UK

Robert C Read
Professor of Infectious Diseases, Section of Infection and Immunity, Division of Molecular and Genetic Medicine, University of Sheffield Medical School, UK

2002 First edition
2005, 2006 Revised and updated edition
2006 Second edition
Published by the Royal Society of Medicine Press Ltd
1 Wimpole Street, London W1G 0AE, UK
Tel: +44 (0) 20 7290 2921
Fax: +44 (0) 20 7290 2929
Email: publishing@rsm.ac.uk
Website: www.rsmpress.co.uk

British Library Cataloguing in Publication Data
A catalogue record for this book is available from the British Library

ISBN 1-85315-698-1
ISSN 1473 6845

Distribution in Europe and Rest of World:
Marston Book Services Ltd
PO Box 269
Abingdon
Oxon OX14 4YN, UK
Tel: +44 (0) 1235 465 500
Fax: +44 (0) 1235 465 555
Email: direct.order@marston.com

Distribution in Australia and New Zealand:
Elsevier Australia
30–52 Smidmore Street
Marrickville NSW 2204
Australia
Tel: + 61 2 9517 8999
Fax: + 61 2 9517 2249
Email: service@elsevier.com.au

Distribution in the USA and Canada:
Royal Society of Medicine Press Ltd
c/o BookMasters, Inc
30 Amberwood Parkway
Ashland, Ohio 44805, USA
Tel: +1 800 247 6553 / +1 800 266 5564
Fax: +1 419 281 6883
E-mail: order@bookmasters.com

Typeset by Phoenix Photosetting, Chatham, Kent
Printed in Europe by the Alden Group, Oxford

About the authors

Roy Jennings is Emeritus Professor in the Section of Infection and Immunity, Division of Genomic Medicine at the University of Sheffield. He graduated in microbiology from the University of Birmingham in 1960, gaining his PhD in 1967 at the University of the West Indies by working on respiratory viral infections. On returning to the UK, he spent five years as a Lecturer in Virology in the Department of Microbiology at the University of Leeds, before moving to the Department of Medical Microbiology at the University of Sheffield Medical School. He was Professor of Virology and Head of Department from 1993 to 1999. His research work has been primarily concerned with the disease of influenza, the influenza viruses and their control. He has published over 90 scientific papers on these topics.

Robert C Read is Professor of Infectious Diseases in the Section of Infection and Immunity, Division of Molecular and Genetic Medicine at the University of Sheffield Medical School, and Honorary Consultant Physician to the Sheffield Teaching Hospitals. He received his medical undergraduate training at the University of Sheffield, and has postgraduate training experience in Leeds, Bristol, London, Nottingham and San Francisco. His research interests include the pathogenesis and prevention of severe infections of the respiratory tract, including influenza.

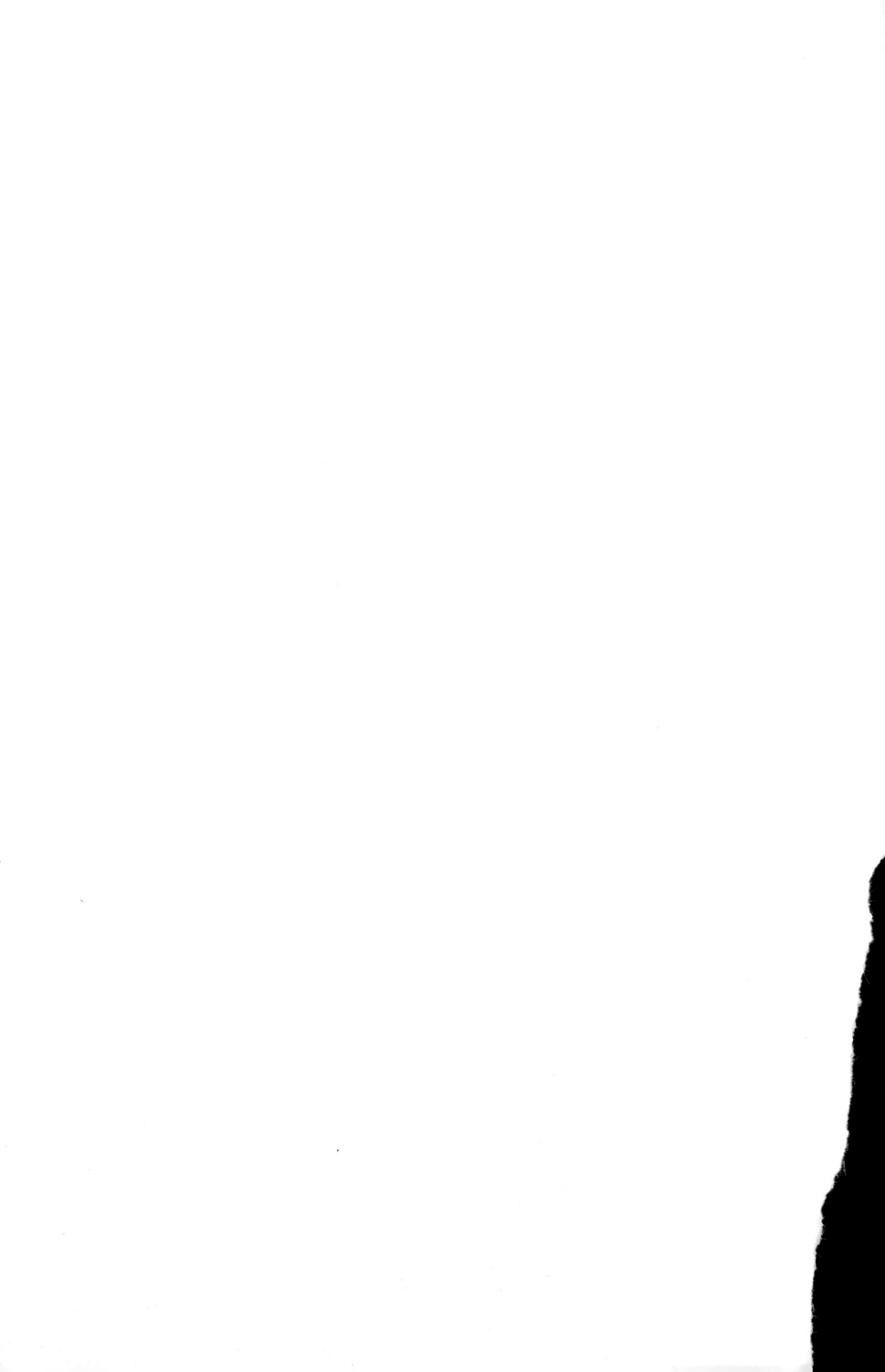

Preface

Influenza is currently under the spotlight for several reasons. In the modern era, where rapid and relatively easy global travel is commonplace, the spread of infectious diseases, particularly those involving transmission via the respiratory tract – and particularly influenza – presents a very real and almost annual threat to communities worldwide. Among the high-density population in the UK, recent epidemics of influenza have caused widespread morbidity, together with extensive levels of mortality in certain risk groups. These widespread outbreaks have sometimes been accompanied by disruption to essential healthcare and other services. The epidemics and outbreaks of influenza have also given rise to considerable adverse publicity, largely directed at the government of the time and its policies, or lack of them, for dealing with such eventualities. The fact that such illness, death and disruption can still occur in a modern society – in spite of the availability of both a vaccine against the infection and an extensive surveillance network to monitor the appearance, the genetic and antigenic make-up, and the spread of influenza virus strains – serves only to illustrate the magnitude of the problem.

A further reason for the current extensive and global interest in influenza lies in the several increasingly common reports of the transmission of a number of avian influenza virus strains to humans and the high morbidity and mortality rates observed in humans unfortunate enough to have been infected by these strains. This increased recent cross-species transmission activity of influenza viruses has been reported not just between avian species and humans, but also between horses and dogs. The reason for this apparently sudden and recent increase in the global activity of the influenza viruses remains unknown, but raises the real and worrying spectre of a new influenza virus pandemic arising in the near future, involving a strain of the virus essentially novel to, and possibly of considerable lethality for, the human population.

Notwithstanding the above, over recent years, a number of important scientific advances in man's ongoing battle with the influenza virus and the disease it causes have given rise to optimism that the annual impact of the disease may be reduced in the near future. Progress in understanding the epidemiology of influenza and its transmission to humans, and the immune mechanisms that underlie the control of the infection, is fuelling both the current development of novel vaccines and the recognition that there could be more effective methods of delivery for these preparations than the conventional intramuscular route. In addition, the past five years have witnessed the advent of a number of drugs that are able to reduce the symptoms of influenza, provided they are administered early enough in the infection.

This book, aimed primarily at medical practitioners working in either the general community or industrial- or company-based practices, should also be found useful by hospital-based consultants, junior doctors, nursing staff and other individuals connected with the healthcare profession. Besides reviewing and updating the biological characteristics of the influenza viruses, the book explains the epidemiological and immune mechanisms that have important roles in, and form the background to, the pathogenesis of influenza infection. Two chapters describe the clinical features of influenza as it presents in different population groups. The current situation with respect to the use of vaccines for immunization against influenza, and the nature and rationale behind the recent development of anti-influenza drugs, constitute a further two chapters. The final chapter is concerned with the management of influenza in general practice.

This second edition covers the new NICE guidelines on the treatment of influenza.

Roy Jennings
Robert C Read

July 2006

Contents

Introduction 1

1 **Nature of the influenza viruses 3**
Structure 3
Growth and replication 4
Variability 5
Nomenclature 6
Influenza viruses in non-human species 6
Type B and C influenza viruses 7

2 **Epidemiology 9**
Infection patterns 9
Antigenic variability in Type A viruses 9
Virulence factors 12
Resistance to infection 12

3 **Pathogenesis 15**
Establishment of infection 15
Pathogenetic effects 16
Role of interferon 17
Role of local host factors 17
Serum antibody 18
Protection and clearance 18

4 **Relationships between avian, mammalian and human influenza viruses 21**
Epidemiology 23
Pathogenicity and virulence 24
Clinical disease in the non-human host 26
Control 27
Cross-species transmission 29

5 **Clinical assessment 31**
Symptoms in adults 31
Symptoms in children 31
Influenza virus pneumonia 32
Diagnosis 33
Influenza in pregnancy 34
Overview of management of seasonal influenza 34
Clinical features of avian influenza 34

6 **Complications and 'at-risk' populations 37**
The immunocompromised patient 37
Secondary bacterial complications 37
Conclusions 40

7 **Immunization 43**
Efficacy 43
Groups recommended for vaccination 43
Vaccine production 44
Safety 46
Problems 46
Determination of vaccine immunogenicity 47
New strategies of vaccination 47
Local and systemic immune mechanisms 48
Novel vaccines 49
Use of vaccines in general practice 49

8 **Antiviral drugs for treatment and prevention 55**
Amantadine and rimantadine 55
Neuraminidase inhibitors 55
Prophylaxis 59

9 **Management 63**
Immunization 63
Diagnosis 63
Standard treatment 65
Complications 66
The workplace 67

Useful websites 69

Index 71

Introduction

The illness that we call influenza, and the viruses responsible for causing this infection, probably date back to antiquity. The 'Great Plague of Athens', dating to about 430–437 BC could have been influenza, although recent DNA examination of ancient dental pulp suggests typhoid fever as a possible cause. Down through the centuries, other descriptions of various outbreaks and epidemics erupting from time to time suggest influenza as a possible cause. In the modern era, it was the devastating pandemic of 1918 – 'Spanish' or 'swine' influenza – that first brought the disease to worldwide public notice. Over the past few years, outbreaks or epidemics of 'seasonal' influenza, of greater or lesser severity, seem to have become a regular feature of life in the UK almost every winter. There is an increased awareness of the medical and economic burdens that have to be shouldered by the community to meet and control infection by these viruses. Influenza infection contributes to a significant annual increase in both morbidity and mortality in the UK during every winter season. It is associated with at least 3000–4000 deaths, primarily in elderly persons suffering from some form of chronic illness. During a substantial epidemic, more than 20 000 excess deaths may occur, and the effects may be compounded by severe disruption to essential services.

In spite of the undoubted community-wide effects of influenza epidemics and outbreaks, there are currently grounds for optimism with regard to improving control of the infection. These are due, in part, to the recent development of several new safe anti-influenza drugs, which have been shown to be efficacious in clinical trials and are now available for use in specific population groups. These novel compounds, which act specifically against the virus, can shorten and ameliorate the clinical symptoms of influenza and also reduce the extent of virus shedding in nasal secretions, thereby showing potential for reducing spread of the virus. Some of these drugs also exhibit some prophylactic potential against influenza virus infection. There is also increasing optimism that progress is being made towards the prevention of influenza through novel vaccination strategies. It is generally agreed that the current commercially available influenza vaccines, although showing a degree of efficacy in reducing morbidity and mortality in certain groups within the population, are less than ideal, particularly in the face of a large-scale epidemic, or a pandemic associated with a novel Type A strain of virus.

The influenza Type A viruses possess the capacity to undergo consistent genetic variation of their nucleic acid, resulting in regular, indeed almost annual, phenotypic modifications and changes in the protein antigens present on their surface. In turn, such alterations in antigenic structure influence the extent of recognition of these proteins by the immune defences of the host when virus infection takes place. This 'trick' is the main means by which the influenza virus has evaded complete control by vaccination until now, despite the considerable efforts of researchers and clinicians since the initial isolation of the virus in 1933. Over the past decade or so, however, burgeoning molecular biology and genetic engineering technology has led to the development of several novel vaccines, produced through the use of clever and complex molecular and genetic strategies, against many different microbial agents. Some of these vaccines have become commercially available for all or specific population groups. There is currently considerable interest and research into the application of these strategies for the further development of influenza vaccines. These novel approaches have been coupled with the parallel development of methodology that will permit effective delivery of such vaccine preparations into the respiratory tract of the human host – the most appropriate site for preventing influenza virus infection. These researches, which have been accompanied by an increased understanding of the nature of the immune mechanisms operating against influenza viruses in the human respiratory tract, suggest that a new generation of such vaccines may become a reality within the next three to five years.

There is an increased awareness of the medical and economic burdens that are shouldered by the community to meet and control infection by influenza viruses.

This book provides an overview of the virological and clinical aspects of influenza. It includes chapters devoted to the pathogenesis of the disease and the interaction of the viruses with host tissues and immune defences, the epidemiology of the infection and its relevance and impact on those groups at greatest risk from the disease, and the current situation with regard to control, treatment and management of the infection through vaccines and anti-influenza drugs. In addition a new chapter has been included, concerned with the epidemiology and disease associated with Type A influenza viruses in avian and non-human mammalian species, and the potential for, and the manner whereby, the spread of these infections into humans may take place.

Further reading

Langmuir AD, Worthen TD, Solomon J *et al.* The Thucydides syndrome. A new hypothesis for the cause of the plague of Athens. *N Engl J Med* 1985; **313**: 1027–30.

Papgrigorakis MJ, Yapijakis C, Synodinos PN *et al.* DNA examination of ancient dental pulp incriminates typhoid fever as a probable cause of the Plague of Athens. *Int J Inf Dis* 2006; **10**: 206–214.

1. Nature of the influenza viruses

Structure
Growth and replication
Variability
Nomenclature
Influenza viruses in non-human species
Type B and C influenza viruses

Influenza viruses are members of the family Orthomyxoviridae, which incorporates three virus types: Types A, B and C. The basis of the difference between these virus types lies in the molecular nature of a major internal protein, the nucleocapsid protein (NP), which surrounds the ribonucleic acid (RNA) gene segments (forming ribonucleoprotein (RNP) structures).

- Types A and B influenza viruses contain eight RNA gene segments.
- Type C influenza virus contains only seven RNA gene segments.

The RNA gene segments of Type A and B viruses code for 11 viral proteins, 3 of which are located on the surface of the mature virus particle (virion). Seven of the remaining proteins are located in the virion interior and have multiple functions concerned with:

- virion integrity
- protection of viral RNA
- translocation of virion components within the host cell
- replication, packaging, assembly and maturation of the virus in the host cell.

Four of these internal proteins – NP itself plus the three P proteins (PB1, PB2 and PA) that make up the polymerase enzyme of the virus – form the structure of the viral nucleocapsid.

Functionally, these proteins form the transcriptase complex. They act in concert and are instrumental in 'kick-starting' virus replication within the infected host cell. Another protein, recently termed the 'nuclear export protein', appears to have the major function of ensuring proper egress of progeny viral nucleocapsids from the host cell nucleus. One other protein, the non-structural protein NS_1, which also contributes to viral replication and the intracellular translocation of virion components, is expressed from the viral genome only in the infected host cell. It has not been found in mature virus particles.

> There are three types of influenza virus: Type A, Type B and Type C

Structure

The basic structure of the influenza virus consists of a central core or 'nucleocapsid' containing most of the internal proteins and the viral RNA segments (Figure 1.1). External to the nucleocapsid, but closely associated and integral with it, is a major structural protein of the virus. This matrix (M_1) protein is primarily responsible for virion integrity. The M_1 protein also interacts with the structure external to it – the lipid envelope of the virus, which carries three important viral glycoproteins. The function of these glycoproteins is to facilitate the entry and exit of the virus into and from the host cell. They project through the lipid envelope and appear as 'spikes' in electron micrographs. The lipids in the envelope of the influenza virus are derived from the host cell. This is because the virus is assembled at and emerges through the cell membrane on completion of its replication cycle.

Mature extracellular influenza virus particles are normally approximately spherical, ranging in size from about 90 to 120 nm in diameter (Fig 1.2).

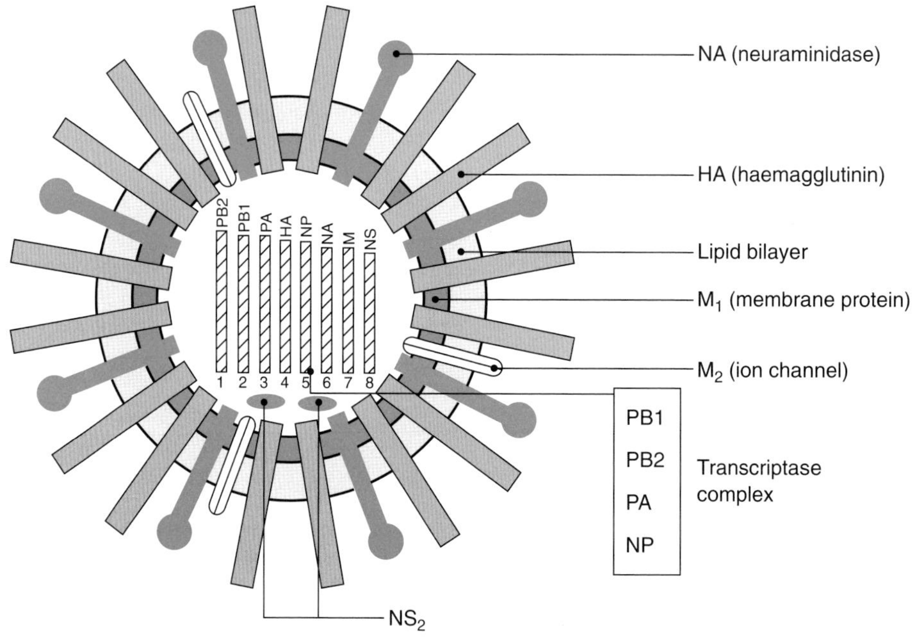

Figure 1.1
Schematic representation of an influenza virus particle. [Reproduced from De Jong JC, Rimmelzwaan CF, Fouchier RA, Osterhaus AD. Influenza virus: a master of metamorphosis. *J Infect* 2000; **40**: 218–28. With kind permission of the publisher WB Saunders.]

Growth and replication

The replication cycle of the virus starts with its attachment to specific receptors on susceptible host cells. In humans, these are usually epithelial cells lining the respiratory passages. These receptors have been identified as the terminal sialic (neuraminic) acid residues on the oligosaccharide side-chains of susceptible cells.

The virus then penetrates the host cell inside an endocytic vesicle, where it is 'uncoated' – the lipid envelope and matrix protein of the particle are degraded by host cell processes. These processes include a marked reduction in the pH inside the endocytic vesicle. The lowered pH also triggers a structural change in the surface haemagglutinin (HA) protein antigen of the virus and exposes the viral nucleocapsid. The nucleocapsid, which contains the viral RNA and several viral proteins with enzymatic functions concerned with viral replication, is unaffected by the low pH. It remains intact, and is released into the cell cytoplasm once the vesicle undergoes natural degradation. The nucleocapsid then migrates to the nucleus of the host cell.

In the nucleus, the viral RNA and the associated viral enzymes direct the formation of messenger RNA for the manufacture of progeny viral proteins in the cell cytoplasm, and progeny viral RNA in the nucleus. Following the relocation of several of these progeny molecules into the nucleus of the host cell and the formation of progeny nucleocapsids, the latter migrate to the cell surface, where they accumulate just beneath the host cell membrane. Other progeny viral molecules, HA and neuraminidase (NA) in particular, migrate through the cell cytoplasm without prior relocation to the nucleus. They are inserted into the host cell membrane, where they project into the surrounding microenvironment. At this

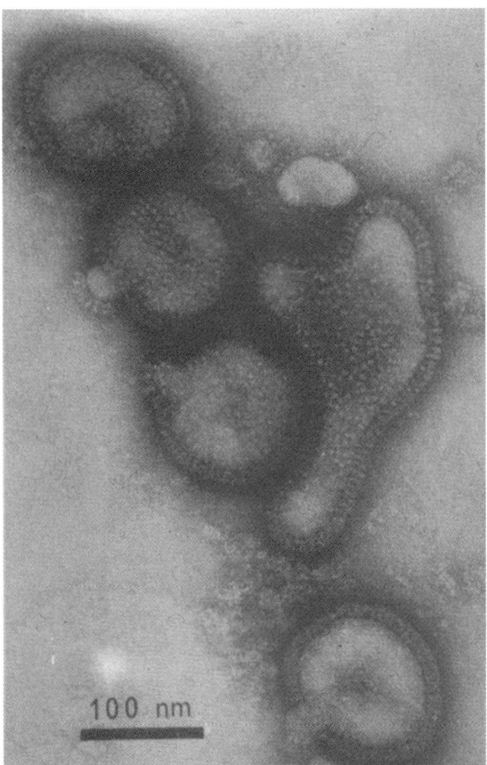

Figure 1.2
Electron micrograph of influenza virus particles. [Reproduced from Emond RTD, Rowland HAK, Welsby PD. A *Colour Atlas of Infectious Diseases*, 3rd edn. London: Wolfe, 1995. With kind permission from Times Mirror International Publishers Ltd.]

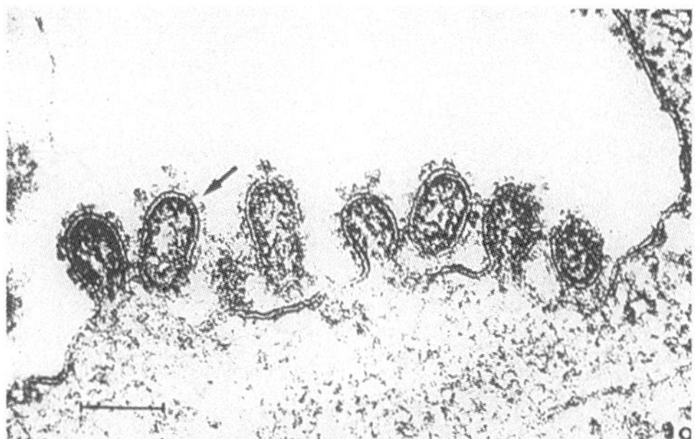

Figure 1.3
Electron micrograph showing influenza virus particles being released from an infected cell by the 'budding' process. The arrow indicates the surface antigen 'spikes' on one of the virus particles. Stained with uranyl acetate and lead citrate (× 100 000).

point, and under the direction of the M_1 protein, maturation of the progeny nucleocapsids and assembly with progeny viral surface proteins embedded in the cell membrane take place. Finally, 'budding' and release of the mature progeny virions occurs by a process termed exocytosis (Figure 1.3). These progeny virions may now infect other, neighbouring, susceptible cells and be shed from the body in the respiratory secretions.

Variability

Although morphologically similar, Types A, B and C influenza viruses exhibit different patterns of epidemiological and clinical behaviour. Type A viruses are associated with most of the widespread influenza epidemics, and are the sole cause of the occasional global pandemics. They have the greatest propensity to cause severe infection, and also predispose to secondary bacterial pneumonia in certain groups of the population. The two most abundant surface glycoproteins of Type A influenza viruses (HA and NA) also show the greatest extent of variability, undergoing subtle, minor changes in structure almost annually. HA and NA are important as targets for the immune defences in controlling influenza virus infection. HA is approximately eight times more abundant on the surface of the virus particle than NA. The minor changes in the structure of these glycoproteins are primarily the consequence of point mutations in the viral RNA genes coding for them. These probably arise because of the absence of a proofreading mechanism to correct mistakes occurring as the virus nucleic acid replicates inside the host cell. This ongoing variability of Type A virus surface proteins is known as 'antigenic drift'. Antigenic drift is the major reason for the success of these viruses in evading human immune mechanisms and causing frequent outbreaks and epidemics.

> Most influenza epidemics are associated with Type A viruses

Figure 1.4 illustrates the regular outbreaks in the UK caused by the influenza viruses over a 12-year period as a consequence of this antigenic drift.

> Type A viruses are associated with most influenza epidemics and are the sole cause of the occasional global pandemics. They can cause severe infection, and also predispose to secondary bacterial pneumonia in certain people. They undergo subtle, minor changes in structure almost annually

Nomenclature

The nomenclature of the influenza viruses that infect humans is derived from four components:

- the virus type (A or B)
- the place where the virus was initially isolated, for example Beijing in China
- the sequential number of the isolate as designated by the World Health Organization Influenza Surveillance Network
- the year of isolation.

Thus A/Beijing/32/92 is a Type A virus isolated in Beijing in 1992.

Influenza viruses in non-human species

Several mammalian and avian species are hosts to Type A influenza viruses that bear genetically similar yet antigenically different versions of the same surface glycoproteins HA and NA as those present on human Type A viruses. Wild avian species are primary reservoirs for Type A influenza viruses. Very occasionally, humans become infected with a virus bearing HA and/or NA antigens derived from non-human sources. These are essentially novel to humans, and this can give rise to a localized outbreak that may develop into a worldwide influenza pandemic. This is because the HA and/or NA surface antigens of such viruses are not initially recognized by the specific human host defence mechanisms. Because the viruses meet with little or no established resistance, they can, following mutation and adaptation to their new host, spread relatively easily in the human species.

> When humans are infected by a novel virus with a non-human origin, a localized outbreak may occur, which could turn into a worldwide pandemic

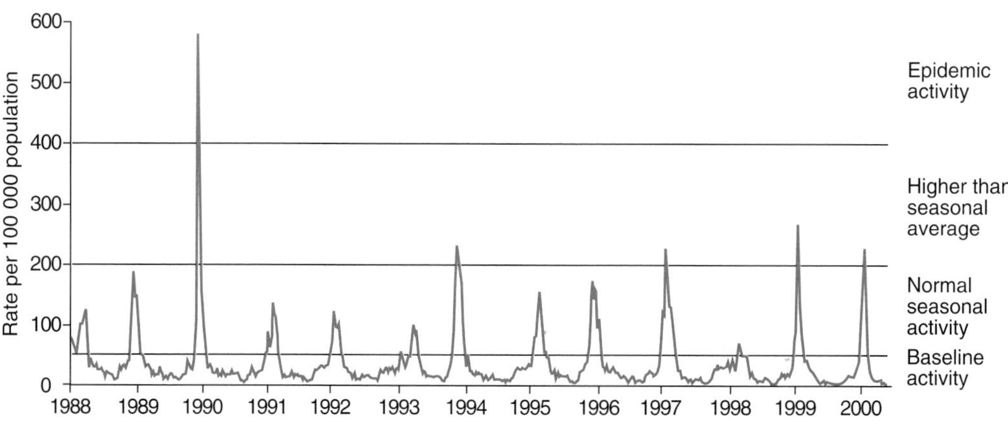

Figure 1.4
Weekly consultation rates for influenza and influenza-like illness. Weekly Returns Service of the Royal College of General Practitioners, 1988–2000. [Adapted from Fleming DM. The contributions of influenza to combined acute respiratory infections, hospital admissions, and deaths in winter. *Commun Dis Public* Health 2000; **3**: 32–8. With kind permission of the PHLS Communicable Disease Surveillance Centre ©PHLS.]

A recent example of this occurred in Hong Kong in 1997, and subsequently in several countries in southeast Asia, when the H5N1 strains of the Type A influenza virus caused some severe and even lethal infections in humans. Fortunately, these outbreaks were effectively contained, and by 2004 the virus had not become established in humans, or adapted to transmission between humans, although further spread of the virus in avian species to other parts of the world has continued since then.

Table 1.1
Nucleotide substitution rates for the haemagglutinin (HA) gene of Type A and Type B influenza viruses

Influenza virus type	*Annual nucleotide substitution rate in gene coding for viral HA glycoprotein (%)*
A	0.40–0.70
B	0.18–0.20

Adapted from Smith DB, Inglis SC. *J Gen Virol* 1987; **68**: 2729–40

Type B and C influenza viruses

In general, Type B influenza viruses cause milder illnesses than Type A viruses. Nevertheless, infection with a Type B virus can range from an illness accompanied by no more than common cold-like symptoms to typical, severe influenza. Symptomatic Type B influenza virus infections are more common in children than in adults. Infections of adults with Type B virus are more often mild or asymptomatic (although occasional severe disease does occur). The frequency of infections with Type B influenza viruses requiring hospitalization is only about one-quarter of that for the Type A viruses.

Although its structure and organization are similar to that of Type A influenza virus, Type B influenza virus has limited variation in the genes coding for its surface HA and NA proteins, and the mutation rate associated with its RNA is lower than that of the Type A virus (Table 1.1). The lower mutation rate and absence of any mammalian or avian reservoir for Type B influenza viruses means that they represent less of a clinical or epidemiological problem than Type A viruses.

Type C influenza virus is associated with only asymptomatic or mild common cold-like illnesses in humans. Both its genome and its protein structure are organized slightly differently from those of the Type A or B viruses, and it undergoes no antigenic variation of its single surface protein.

The influenza viruses have been recorded as causing infections, outbreaks, epidemics and pandemics in humans from ancient times, and the disease has been considered to be one of the last great uncontrolled plagues of humankind. However, recent advances in both chemoprophylaxis and chemotherapy for the infection indicate that some progress is being made in combating this disease.

> Influenza may be considered to be one of the last great uncontrolled plagues of humankind

Further reading

Ellis J, Joseph C, Zambon M. Fifty years of influenza serveillance. *Commun Dis Public Health* 1999; **2**: 81–2.

Ellis J, Zambon M. Strain designation for influenza viruses. *Commun Dis Public Health* 1999; **2**: 157–9.

Potter CW. A history of influenza. J Appl Microbiol 2001; **91**: 572–9.

Ruigrok, RWH. Structure of influenza A, B and C viruses. In: Nicholson KG, Webster RG, Hay AJ (eds). *Textbook of Influenza*. Oxford: Blackwell, 1998.

Smith DB, Inglis SC. The mutation rate and variability of eukaryotic viruses: an analytical review. *J Gen Virol* 1987; **68**: 2729–40.

2. Epidemiology

Infection patterns
Antigenic variability in Type A viruses
Virulence factors
Resistance to infection

Because influenza viruses possess a lipid envelope, they are relatively labile. They can only survive in an infectious form on inert surfaces outside the human or animal host for short periods of time. Their survival time is also dependent on the presence of accompanying proteinaceous material. Several carefully conducted studies carried out in the 1980s indicated that the half-life of Type A influenza virus particles in saline on an inert surface in the absence of any protein is approximately 2–3 hours. However, in the presence of high concentrations of protein, the half-life rises to about 4–6 hours. Because of these findings, it is generally believed that most human influenza virus infections are transmitted through direct transfer of aerosols or droplets carrying the virus from the respiratory tract of one person to that of another.

> Most human influenza virus infections are spread through aerosols or droplets carrying the virus

Infection patterns

The incubation period for influenza virus infections are:

- 3 days for Type A virus
- 4 days for Type B virus.

Viral replication in the respiratory tract of normal adults peaks approximately 48 hours after infection. Progeny virions are shed in nasal secretions and saliva from about 1 to 7 days after infection (Figure 2.1). Children of preschool and school age are major vectors for influenza virus transmission. In these children, the virus is shed from day 1 postinfection and may still be present up to day 13 postinfection.

Antigenic variability in Type A viruses

A major characteristic of influenza viruses, particularly Type A viruses, is the antigenic variability of their surface haemagglutinin (HA) and neuraminidase (NA) proteins.

Antigenic drift

Antigenic drift occurs in both of the surface proteins, although it is greatest for HA. It is a virtually ongoing process, resulting from spontaneous point mutations occurring in the viral genes coding for these proteins as the virus replicates in the human body. These mutations are manifest at the phenotypic level as distinct alterations in the reactivity of the surface proteins every 2–3 years. The manifestations are seen only when the accumulated effect of a series of point mutations becomes detectable by laboratory methods. The changes in the surface protein structure of strains recently isolated from humans can be observed in the laboratory through the altered interaction of their HA or NA with specific antibodies to the HA or NA of existing, previously isolated strains.

> Most antigenic variation is seen in the HA protein, although the NA protein also undergoes antigenic drift

The antigenic changes are responsible for the reduced capacity of any pre-existing antibody to previously experienced influenza virus to combine with and hence effectively neutralize the altered virus strain. The net result of these mutations is an imperfect match between the antigen present on the current virus and the

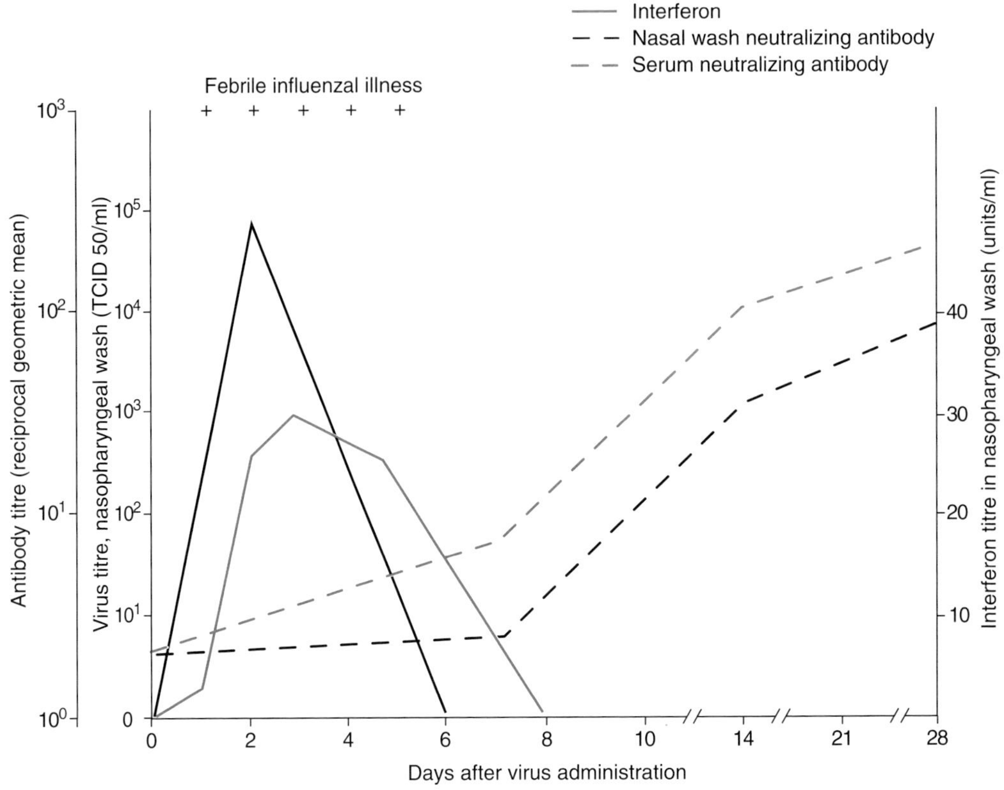

Figure 2.1
Mean patterns of virus titre, serum and nasal wash antibody levels, febrile response, and nasal wash interferon levels over time in six seronegative volunteers given 104.0 tissue culture infectious doses of wild-type A/Hong Kong/68-like virus intranasally on day 0. (TCID, tissue culture infectious dose.) [Reproduced from Murphy BR, Webster RG. Orthomyxoviruses. In: Fields BN, Knipe DM, Chanock RM *et al.* (eds) *Fields' Virology*, 2nd edn. Philadelphia: Raven Press, 1990: 1091–152.]

pre-existing antibody induced in response to contact with earlier strains of the virus. This inefficient neutralizing action of the antibody permits a more effective uptake of the modified virus by susceptible cells and therefore a greater probability for the establishment of infection.

Antigenic shift

Laboratory evidence indicates that the 20th century saw five influenza pandemics resulting from the appearance of a Type A virus bearing an HA protein that was essentially novel to the contemporary human population. The best known of these was the pandemic of 1918 – the 'swine' or 'Spanish' influenza epidemic – which reportedly caused in excess of 20 million deaths, primarily in young adults. The most recent, but much less devastating, pandemic occurred in 1977. It saw the reappearance of a virus with HA having similarities to that responsible for the 1918 pandemic, and also to that involved in the pandemic of 1933–34.

Almost all of these sudden major changes in the Type A influenza surface antigens initially occurred in China. A number of these 'new' influenza viruses have arisen by genetic reassortment between human and either mammalian or avian influenza viruses bearing different surface proteins. Genetic reassortment has been detected *in vivo* in both humans and animal species. Such reassortment is dependent on the random distribution of the genomic material of two distinct Type A influenza viruses present and undergoing replication in the same cell. In general, the different Type A influenza virus subtypes infect only a single host species. When the occasional cross-species transmission of a subtype occurs however, genetic reassortment can take place in the cells of the new host between the transmitted subtype and a Type A influenza virus of a different subtype already present in that recipient host. This can produce an essentially novel virus bearing surface proteins derived from either parent subtype. Continued replication of this virus in the host can produce further minor modifications of either or both of the surface proteins that may also contribute to its distinct antigenic profile. This virus may now have acquired the capability to become established and transmitted in the new host, or even to be able to infect, establish itself in and be transmitted between individuals of a third host, such as humans.

> Each Type A influenza virus subtype usually only infects one host species

Laboratory studies have unequivocally demonstrated that both the 1957 and the 1968 Type A influenza pandemic strains appeared through genetic reassortment. The 1957 'Asian' influenza virus obtained the two genes coding for its HA and NA surface proteins from an avian Type A influenza virus, together with a gene coding for one of its internal proteins. The remaining five genes present in the Asian Type A virus were all derived from the preceding human Type A influenza virus strain, which had been circulating in the human population since 1933–34.

Across all animal species and in humans, there are 15 different HA proteins (H1,...H15) and 9 different NA proteins (N1,...N9) (a possible 16th HA protein has been identified in a virus isolated from a black-headed gull). To date, only 3 of the HA proteins (H1, H2 and H3) have been found in those Type A influenza viruses that are able to infect and become established in humans. Over the past 8 years, there have been several small, yet clinically severe, outbreaks of Type A influenza in various parts of the world. These outbreaks have been caused by viruses bearing non-human haemagglutinin H5, H7 or H9 antigens. The viruses responsible are from domestic poultry sources, and their transmission to humans is covered in more detail in Chapter 4.

The severity of this infection in apparently healthy individuals aged 13–60 years was of considerable concern, creating a new awareness of the direct infective potential of avian influenza viruses for humans. Nevertheless, this virus did not spread from one patient to another, and did not therefore become established in humans.

Since the pandemic of 1977 (known as 'Russian flu' on account of its origin from a laboratory somewhere in the former Soviet Union), two Type A influenza virus subtypes have been circulating among humans worldwide. These subtypes are:

- the H1N1 virus – Russian 'flu
- the H3N2 subtype – which first appeared in the population in 1968 as the cause of the 'Hong Kong' pandemic.

Both viruses have been undergoing antigenic drift since their first appearance in the human population. Since 1977, there has been no introduction, spread or establishment of a novel Type A influenza virus on a global scale. The duration and years of prevalence of the various Type A influenza subtypes that have circulated in humans from 1918 to the present time are listed in Table 2.1.

> The current Type A influenza virus subtypes circulating in humans are H3N2 and H1N1

Table 2.1
Subtypes of Type A influenza viruses found in humans

Subtype	*Popular name of subtype*	*Years of prevalence*
H1N1 ('swine'-like)	Spanish or swine 'flu	1917–32
H1N1	None	1933–56
H2N2	Asian influenza	1957–67
H3N2	Hong Kong 'flu	1968 – present[a]
H1N1	Russian 'flu	1977 – present[a]

[a] Subtype currently circulating in humans

Virulence factors

The inherent virulence of a given strain of Type A influenza virus remains something of an enigma. Well-defined virulence factors are associated with certain Type A viruses that infect domestic poultry, and such highly virulent strains often cause severe mortality and morbidity at considerable economic cost to the poultry industry. The relevance and importance in humans of the major virulence factor that appears most closely associated with the catastrophic epidemics in poultry does not seem to play a similarly major role in human infection. This property, the cleavability of the linkage site between the two elements, HA_1 and HA_2, of the viral HA by host proteins, is undoubtedly of importance in the pathogenicity of Type A influenza viruses for humans, but a number of other, recently recognized, virulence factors may also be of considerable importance in facilitating high viral virulence and pathogenicity in the human population.

The inherent virulence of any given Type A influenza virus strain is multifactorial, but one factor that may well contribute to this virulence is the non-structural (NS_1) protein. Among its roles in the cell biology of the virus, NS_1 can effectively inhibit the production of interferon-induced antiviral proteins by host cells. These proteins have important roles in the cellular control of influenza and of many other viral infections. NS_1 can also downregulate apoptosis (programmed cell death) in cells infected by Type A viruses. The quality or quantity of functional NS_1 protein produced during infection by a given strain of Type A influenza virus may therefore influence the capacity of that strain to elicit a more or less severe infection.

There have been one or two reports that both the infection rate and the severity of the associated influenzal illness is greater for the H3N2 strains than for the H1N1 strains in humans. The factors that may play a role in these differences remain to be determined.

Resistance to infection

Humans acquire resistance to the influenza virus when they have circulating antibodies to the HA and NA surface proteins of the virus. These antigens project through the lipid envelope of the virus and are also expressed at the surface of infected host cells. Infected cells and virions themselves therefore represent important targets for the immune defence mechanisms of the host. In the human (or animal) host, infection with the influenza viruses elicits:

- a humoral immune response
- a cellular immune response.

The humoral element of this immune response is long-lived in the circulation and is specific for the infecting subtype of influenza virus, ie Type A or Type B. In nature, however, the antigenic drift shown by Type A influenza viruses means that the full effect of this immunity wanes over time. Its duration at protective levels is dependent on the extent of the antigenic change accumulated by the surface proteins (particularly the HA antigen of the virus). Systemic antibody levels to HA have been correlated with protection against influenza virus infection. The role of local, nasal and respiratory tract antibody is increasingly being recognized as an important contributor to the host's defences against this infection.

Influenza virus-specific cell-mediated immune mechanisms, particularly that due to cytotoxic T lymphocytes, play a major role in recovery from infection by influenza viruses. This is probably through the destruction of influenza virus-infected cells in the respiratory tract. This cellular immune mechanism does not become effective until 2 or 3 days after the initial infection. It is more independent of the antigenic variability of the viral surface proteins than the humoral immune response, but is relatively short-lived and lasts for only a few weeks.

> The humoral immune response to an influenza infection is more long lasting than the cell-mediated response, which is only effective for a few weeks

Further reading

Bush RM, Bender CA, Subbarao, K *et al.* Predicting the evolution of human influenza A. *Science* 1999; **286**: 1921–25.

De Jong JC, Rimmelzwaan GF, Fouchier RAM, Osterhaus ADME. Influenza virus: a master of metamorphosis. *J Infect* 2000; **40**: 218–28.

Fields BN, Knipe DM, Chanock RM *et al* (eds). *Fields' Virology,* 2nd edn, Vol 1. Philadelphia: Raven Press, 1990: 1091–152.

Fleming DM. The contribution of influenza to combined acute respiratory infections, hospital admissions, and deaths in winter. *Commun Dis Public Health* 2000; **3**: 32–8.

Ito T, Couceiro JN, Kelm S *et al.* Molecular basis for the generation in pigs of influenza A viruses with pandemic potential. *J Virol* 1998; **72**: 7367–73.

Mortimer P. On being prepared: the Influenza Pandemic Plan. *Common Dis Public Health* 2001; **4**: 156–7.

Murphy BR, Webster RG. Orthomyxoviruses. In: Fields BN, Knipe DM, Chanock RM *et al.* (eds) *Fields' Virology*, 2nd edn. Philadelphia: Raven Press, 1990: 1091–152.

Nguyen-Van-Tam JS. Epidemiology of influenza. In: Nicholson KG, Webster RG, Hay AJ (eds). *Textbook of Influenza.* Oxford: Blackwell, 1998.

Pickrell J. The 1918 pandemic. Killer flu with a human–pig pedigree. *Science* 2001; **292**: 1041.

Simonsen L. The global impact of influenza on morbidity and mortality. *Vaccine* 1999; **17** Suppl 1: S3–10.

Webster RG, Bean WJ, Gorman OT et al. Evolution and ecology of influenza A viruses. *Microbiol Rev* 1992; **56**: 152–79.

Zhirnov OP, Konakova TE, Wolff T, Klenk HD. NS1 protein of influenza A virus down-regulates apoptosis. *J Virol* 2002; **76**: 1617–25.

3. Pathogenesis

Establishment of infection
Pathogenetic effects
Role of interferon
Role of local host factors
Serum antibody
Protection and clearance

Influenza viruses are transmitted not only via droplet spread in nasal secretions and saliva (expelled particularly during coughing and sneezing), but also during the ordinary daily contact of humans with each other. Particles generated during coughing or sneezing are usually less than 2 nm in diameter. Particles of this size are normally deposited in the lower airways of the lung.

Establishment of infection

The stages of infection with a Type A influenza virus depend on contact of the inhaled virus with susceptible mucosal epithelial cells in the human respiratory tract. This contact allows attachment of the virus to its specific cellular receptors. It is suggested that most successful influenza virus infections are established in the lower respiratory tract. However, this does not necessarily preclude the possibility that a significant number may be initiated in the nasal passages of the upper respiratory tract.

It is also becoming increasingly recognized that an infection is more likely to be successfully established where influenza-specific antibodies, particularly local immunoglobulin A (IgA), are either absent altogether or present at only low levels in the respiratory tract. In the presence of local antibodies, the attachment of influenza virus particles to their specific host cell receptors will be inhibited. The antibody can also attach to the viral surface proteins, particularly haemagglutinin (HA), and block the activity of the virus particles.

> Most successful influenza virus infections are probably established in the lower respiratory tract

Factors influencing establishment of infection

The closeness of the match between the incoming virus and any existing local antibodies is particularly important when establishing an infection. The presence of local antibodies to Type B influenza, however high their level, will not influence the establishment of a Type A influenza virus infection. Similarly, due to the phenomenon of antigenic drift shown annually by Type A influenza viruses, the presence of antibodies to a strain of influenza A virus encountered 3 or 4 years previously may have only a limited effect in preventing establishment of infection by a current Type A strain. Following establishment of the virus, there may be a very transient viraemia, but it is generally not possible to recover virus from the bloodstream of infected individuals. Similarly, there is no unequivocal evidence that the virus can persist or exist in any latent form in the human host.

The ability of the influenza viruses to establish infection in humans will thus be dependent on:

- several nonspecific and virus-specific host factors
- viral factors, such as the quantity of virus inhaled or taken into the respiratory tract
- the intrinsic virulence of the virus.

The greater the amount of virus taken into the respiratory tract, the greater the chance the virus has of overcoming any local specific, extracellular defence mechanisms (particularly local antibody). It is also more likely that the virus will attach to and penetrate susceptible mucosal columnar epithelial cells. As part of the non-specific defences of the host, the mucociliary escalator will remove a proportion of the invading virus particles. This is most effective in healthy non-smoking individuals.

> The ability of influenza virus to establish infection depends on various host factors, the quantity of virus in the respiratory tract and how virulent the particular virus strain is

Pathogenetic effects

The lytic replication cycle of the virus commences as soon as it enters a cell. After about 5 or 6 hours, this results in the release of progeny virus particles, which spread gradually to other susceptible cells. In humans, this ultimately results in almost total destruction of the ciliated epithelial cells of the respiratory tract. Similar effects can be observed in ferrets and mice – both of which are good models for human influenza virus infection (Fig 3.1). In both the mouse and ferret, regeneration of the ciliated cells is underway by 7–10 days from the start of infection.

Destruction of epithelial cells

Influenza virus infection in the human nasopharynx results in a loss of the ciliated epithelial cells in this area and also in the trachea (Figure 3.2). These cells are an important element of the human non-specific respiratory tract defences. A major consequence of their destruction is to pave the way for secondary invasion of the lower respiratory tract by bacteria, such as *Streptococcus pneumoniae*, *Staphylococcus aureus* and *Haemophilus influenzae*. This can lead to severe or even fatal pneumonia, particularly in the elderly and other high-risk groups. Bronchoscopy of individuals with uncomplicated influenza virus infection shows the bronchi, trachea and larynx to be:

- deciliated
- oedematous
- acutely inflamed.

The cells are then desquamated.

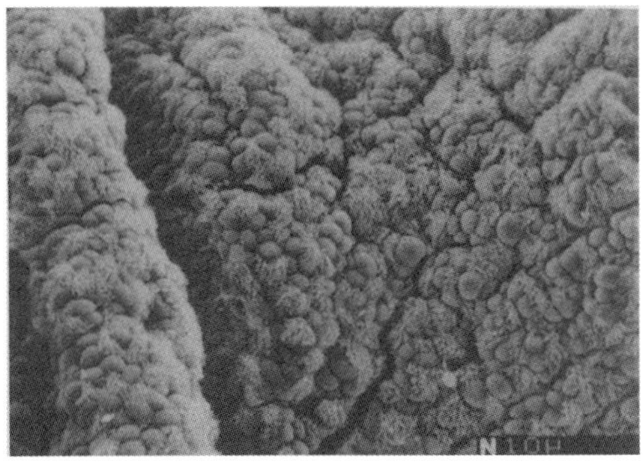

(a)

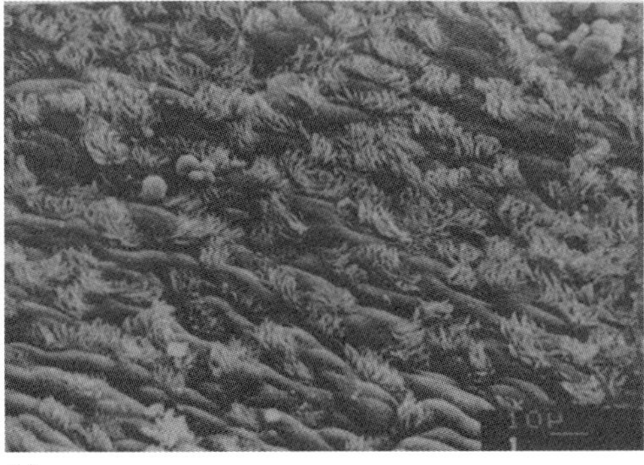

(b)

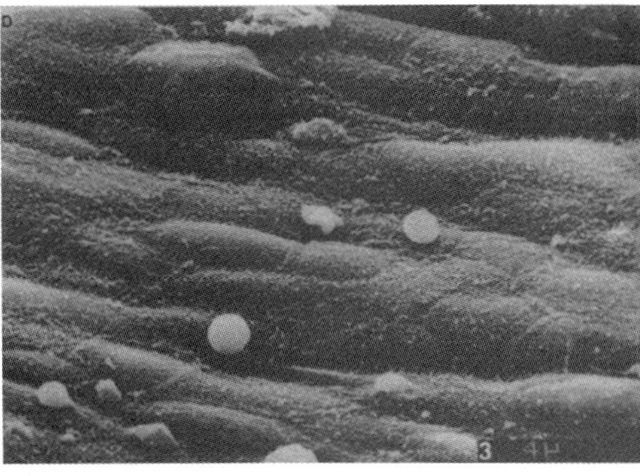

(c)

Figure 3.1
Scanning electron micrographs of (a) normal mouse tracheal epithelium (× 1050), (b) mouse tracheal epithelium 24 hours after infection with Type A virus, showing partial destruction of the ciliated nasal epitheial cells (× 800), and (c) the same cells 72 hours postinfection, showing complete destruction of the cells (× 2000). [Reproduced from Ramphal *et al. American Review of Respiratory Diseases* 1979; **120**: 1313–24.]

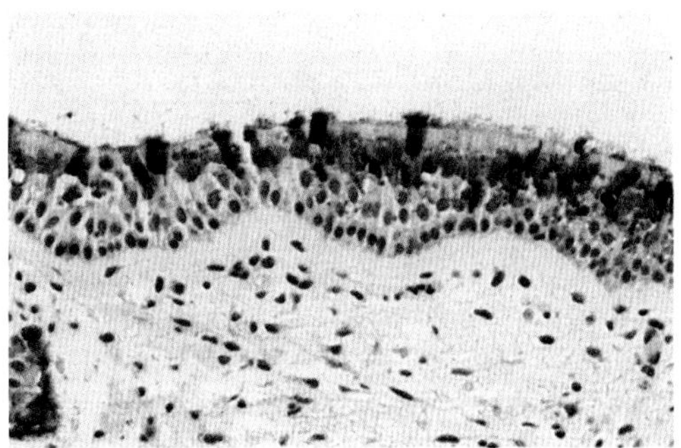

Figure 3.2
Histopathological appearance of human nasopharyngeal explant collected 3 days after the onset of Type B influenza infection. Staining is by an immunoperoxidase method using a polyclonal sheep anti-influenza serum. There is patchy uptake of virus in the epithelial cells, which will ultimately exfoliate.

> Influenza infection results in almost total destruction of the ciliated epithelial cells of the respiratory tract, which paves the way for secondary bacterial infections

Role of interferon

Infection of humans by the influenza viruses probably promotes the full repertoire of the immune and non-immune (non-specific) responses of the host. However, the viruses appear to trigger the interferon (IFN) response of the host extremely effectively. Moreover, there is a direct correlation between the quantities of IFN released from the host's infected cells and the extent of virus replication. IFN is first detected in both the upper respiratory tract secretions and the blood of infected individuals when the clinical symptoms of influenza commence. IFN levels reach a peak about 24 hours later. The cytokine almost certainly plays an important role in reducing replication and limiting spread of the virus in the respiratory tract of the host.

There has been some evidence to show that the clinical symptoms of influenza, particularly the systemic symptoms of malaise, aching back and joints and high temperature, are associated with high levels of IFN. These symptoms are also possibly associated with other proinflammatory cytokines such as interleukin-6 (IL-6) and tumour necrosis factor (TNF). TNF-α has recently been reported to possess stronger anti-influenza virus activity than other cytokines present in human nasal lavage specimens.

Role of local host factors

Other non-specific host factors that play a part in the control of influenza virus infection include:

- soluble factors, such as lung surfactants
- sialylglycoproteins
- alveolar macrophages.

All of these can react with or take up influenza virus particles. Such reactions thereby prevent these virus particles from attaching to and invading the susceptible columnar epithelial cells of the respiratory tract. Another prime factor in controlling infection by influenza viruses is the presence at the time of infection of influenza virus-specific local and systemic antibodies.

Local antibody response

During a primary influenza virus infection (ie one occurring in a host who has never experienced infection by an influenza virus in the past), IgA, IgG and IgM antibodies specific for the viral HA antigen can be detected in nasal washings collected 24–48 hours after the onset of symptoms. The IgA antibodies are actively secreted locally. The IgG antibodies are almost certainly derived from the transudate that spills into the respiratory tract secretions from the bloodstream as a consequence of the inflammatory changes taking place in the nasopharynx as the infection progresses. Both IgA and IgG are capable of neutralizing the virus by preventing its attachment to, or entry into, susceptible columnar epithelial cells. This is done through attaching to the virus particles, thereby blocking the activities of the

HA protein, which is the prime mediator of these viral functions.

There is immunological memory for the local IgA response stimulated following a primary (and a secondary) infection. This is specific for the HA and NA antigens present on the surface of the infecting virus. Changes in the antigenic structure of these proteins through either antigenic drift or antigenic shift reduce or eliminate the capacity of the local IgA to neutralize a different strain of the virus.

Serum antibody

The level of serum antibody, primarily IgG, has been clearly shown to correlate with protection against influenza virus infection. This is only true if there is a close match between the existing antibody and the infecting strain of the virus.

> IgG levels correlate with protection against influenza virus infection

In 80% of naturally acquired influenza virus infections, a systemic IgG antibody response can be demonstrated. With the virus essentially confined to the respiratory tract, it is unclear how systemic IgG reaches the target virus. It has already been stated that in the nasal secretions of humans infected with the Type A influenza virus, there is a preponderance of locally secreted IgA. Also, the concentration of IgG in the nasal wash has been reported to be 350 times less than that in the serum of infected individuals. However, it has been proposed that the observed protective efficacy of systemic anti-influenza IgG is due to the relatively high levels of IgG (compared with IgA) transudated from the circulation into the secretions that bathe the lower respiratory tract. This suggests that most cases of human influenza infection are actually initiated in the lower, rather than the upper, regions of the respiratory tract. There is evidence that this may be the case. Nevertheless, it is likely that a significant proportion of influenza infections are either initiated solely in the upper respiratory tract or arise as a result of invasion of both the upper and lower regions of the respiratory tract. This would therefore provide an explanation for the importance of local IgA in protection against infection by these viruses (Table 3.1).

Protection and clearance

Protection against influenza virus infection is primarily effected through humoral immune mechanisms. The importance of cell-mediated immunity in the early stages of infection is minimal. As already mentioned, the major roles of cellular immune mechanisms are in limiting the spread of an already-established infection and in clearance of the virus from the body through the destruction of infected

Table 3.1
Correlation of HA antibody status with infection in groups of volunteers infected with Type A influenza virus

Antibody status of group				
Serum antibody	*Nasal wash antibody*	*Total No. in group*	*No. infected*	*% infected*
Absent	Absent	16	10	62
Absent	Present	1	0	0
Present	Absent	12	4	33
Present	Present	6	1	17

Adapted from Betts RF, Treanor JJ. Approaches to improved influenza vaccinations. *Vaccine* 2000; **18**: 1690–95. With kind permission from Excerpta Medica Inc.

cells. These activities lead to elimination of the virus from the host and termination of the infection.

Influenza virus infections are eliminated in the host through the action of the cell-mediated immune system

Further reading

Anderson PJ. Factors promoting pathogenicity of influenza virus. *Semin Respir Infect* 1991; **6**: 3–10

Bender BS, Small PA. Influenza: pathogenesis and host defense. *Semin Respir Infect* 1992; **7**: 38–45

Seo SH, Webster RG. Tumor necrosis factor alpha exerts powerful anti-influenza virus effects in lung epithelial cells. *J Virol* 2002; **76**: 1071–6

4. Relationships between avian, mammalian and human influenza viruses

Epidemiology
Pathogenicity and virulence
Clinical disease in the non-human host
Control
Cross-species transmission

Type A influenza viruses are widespread in nature, and many wild and domesticated avian and mammalian species are hosts to Type A, but not to Type B or C, influenza viruses. The Type A influenza viruses of animals and birds are structurally and genetically similar to the Type A viruses infecting humans, and also bear surface glycoproteins – haemagglutinin (HA) and neuraminidase (NA) – that, although antigenically varied, possess functions identical to those of the human viruses. However, there are important differences between these surface proteins at the molecular level, which may influence their epidemiological behaviour and facilitate cross-species transmission.

Wild avian species, particularly aquatic waterfowl and wading birds, represent primary reservoirs for Type A influenza viruses, and these avian Type A viruses spread – probably not infrequently – to other non-human hosts, including domestic poultry such as chickens, ducks and turkeys. Both in the past and recently, transmission of the avian viruses has occurred from domesticated species to humans. Wild waterfowl, gulls and wading birds represent a large, stable, ever-present and highly mobile source of Type A influenza viruses that may regularly seed these viruses into other avian and mammalian species. Indeed, there is high potential for cross-species transfer between animal species, and from animals, including birds, to humans in view of the worldwide interactions between humans, birds, pigs and other mammalian species, and it is perhaps surprising that such interspecies transmission is not documented more frequently.

Interspecies transmission of Type A influenza viruses has a special significance in that within the cells of individual animals or humans that may be coincidentally infected with two serotypes of an influenza virus (or indeed infected with two different strains of the same serotype of influenza virus), there is an opportunity for genetic reassortment between viral genes because of the segmented nature of the Type A viral genome. This is the phenomenon termed antigenic shift, and can give rise to influenza viruses that may be essentially novel to the species, including humans, in which they may arise. This is in addition to the inevitability of mutations occurring over time in the highly mutable genes of the virus, particularly those coding for the HA and NA surface proteins – the process called antigenic drift.

In total, 15 different Type A influenza HA antigens (or 16 if a recently reported novel HA found in a virus isolated from a black-headed gull is confirmed) and 9 NA antigens are known to exist in mammalian and avian species in nature. All of these HA antigens have been isolated from wild or domestic birds, and are listed in Table 4.1. Up to the present time, only Type A influenza serotypes H1, H2 and H3 have been found to be capable of spreading between humans and causing epidemics and pandemics, although viral strains bearing other HA serotypes are clearly able to infect humans. Each of the 9 NA serotypes of Type A influenza virus have also been isolated from wild or domestic birds, but only serotypes bearing the N1 and N2 antigens have so far been found to be transmissible between humans and to be involved in epidemics or pandemics in humans.

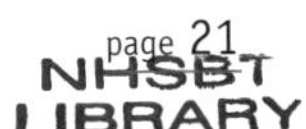

Table 4.1
Type A influenza serotypes found in mammalian and avian species

Haemagglutinin
- All serotypes, H1,...,H15, are found in wild and/or domestic birds
- Serotypes H1 and H3 circulate in pigs
- Serotypes H3 and H7 circulate in horses
- Pilot whales are naturally infected with H13N9 or H13N2 Type A influenza serotypes
- Harbour seals are naturally infected with the H7N7 Type A influenza serotype
- Only serotypes H1, H2 and H3 are so far known to be transmissible between humans

Neuraminidase
- All serotypes, N1,...,N9, are found in wild and/or domestic birds
- Serotypes N1 and N2 are found in pigs
- Serotypes N7 and N8 circulate in horses
- Only serotypes N1 and N2 are so far known to be transmissible between humans

The catastrophic pandemic of 1918 – 'Spanish' or 'swine' influenza – which was reportedly responsible for approximately 20 – 40 million human deaths worldwide, was caused by a Type A influenza virus that was able to spread very rapidly and effectively between humans, and also to spread rapidly and cause severe clinical disease in pigs. However, the origins of this highly virulent virus remain obscure, and it is controversial as to whether the virus appeared and caused illness initially in pigs or in humans. Transfer of Type A influenza viruses from pigs to humans, and from humans to pigs, has been documented on several occasions over the past 30 years, demonstrating that such transmissions between the two species occur in nature.

Since 1997, there have been a series of cross-species transmission events worldwide, involving not pigs in these instances, but domestic birds. So far, several serotypes of Type A influenza viruses having antigenically different combinations of surface HA and NA proteins (H5N1, H9N2, H7N7 and H7N3) have spread by direct transfer from domestic poultry to humans. The H5N1 strains in particular appear to be highly virulent for both poultry and humans, and have exhibited the capacity to cause severe illness and even death in a proportion of affected humans, although they also give rise to asymptomatic human infections. Since 2004, the H5N1 strains of Type A influenza have been responsible for the highest number of human cases of avian influenza ever recorded. However, at the time of writing, humans remain essentially 'dead-end' hosts for these viruses, and there is no evidence that they have acquired the ability to spread easily, effectively or widely in the human species. Nevertheless, there have been a few reports, based on the isolation of H5N1 viruses and the detailed gene sequencing of these strains, together with epidemiological and clinical evidence, indicating that these strains have shown very limited spread between humans via household and social contacts, and, on occasion, have given rise to severe and lethal disease under these circumstances. The scientific community is generally of the opinion that such human-to-human transmission may well happen to a considerably greater extent in the not too distant future as the virus mutates and adapts to existence in the human host, and this might well result in the development of a pandemic caused by these H5N1 viruses.

Further evidence of recent Type A influenza virus interspecies activity was reported in 2004, when it was found that the H5N1 avian influenza virus had spread into tigers and leopards. Two outbreaks in these felines were reported in zoos in Thailand. Type A influenza, serotype H5N1, was recovered from nasal swabs collected from sick tigers, and a number of the animals died. It is probable that the majority of the felines became infected through feeding on the carcasses of chickens infected with this virus, but there is also evidence indicating that transmission of the H5N1 serotype occurred horizontally between tigers as these outbreaks progressed. Although such infection has not been reported in the wild, domestic cats can also be infected by the H5N1 Type A influenza serotype experimentally, via infected chicken carcasses. The cats suffer respiratory symptoms, secrete the virus and can transmit the infection horizontally.

In addition to cross-species transfer of H5N1 Type A influenza strains from poultry into humans and felines, reports in 2003 indicated that another Type A influenza serotype had also crossed the species barrier, in this case from horses into dogs. The first recognized severe clinical outbreak of a disease in canines caused by an influenza virus was recorded in 22 racing greyhounds in Florida in January 2004. Between then, and May 2005, there were 20 further outbreaks of canine influenza at greyhound racetracks in the USA. The Type A influenza virus concerned in these outbreaks has been classified as subtype H3N8, and is virtually identical in its nucleic acid sequence to the H3N8 Type A equine influenza virus that has been present in horses since at least the mid 1960s. Detailed phylogenetic analyses of the viruses involved indicate that a single direct interspecies transmission from horses to dogs has occurred in the recent past. However, mutations in the HA molecule of the virus have occurred, presumably since the interspecies transfer, suggesting that the virus is adapting to its new host. The virus is spreading rapidly among dogs, and is capable of causing severe respiratory illness in these animals. Of the 22 greyhounds infected in the Florida outbreak, 8 died as a result of the infection. Antibody studies demonstrate that there has been spread of this H3N8 virus into pet dogs, suggesting that the virus may become enzootic in these animals. However, the outbreak poses no threat to humans at present.

This increased activity of Type A influenza viruses worldwide may indicate that some rapid evolutionary process has taken place in these viruses over the past few years, perhaps in response to the grouping of animals in captivity, more frequent bulk movements of animals, changes in animal husbandry practices and ever-increasing human travel. Alternatively, the more frequent detection of Type A influenza virus serotypes in non-human species may represent a raised awareness of the importance of influenza in such species and the relevance of this activity to human disease, coupled with the effective and expanding technology available facilitating a more widespread, efficient and successful surveillance for influenza viruses in non-human species.

Up to 2004, the H5N1 Type A avian influenza virus serotype had been transmitted across to humans from domestic poultry in a number of countries in Southeast Asia, but towards the latter half of 2005, such transmission was recorded in Turkey, indicating increased globalization of the virus, although transmission between humans still remains extremely limited.

Epidemiology

Wild waterfowl can transmit Type A influenza viruses via faecal material excreted into water, and many wild birds are infected by virus present in the water of lakes, reservoirs and ponds. It has been estimated that about 30% of wild ducks in North America may excrete virus into the water at the start of the autumn migrations, and it is highly probable that faecal transmission during migration is the means whereby wild ducks spread virus to other wild birds as well as to domestic fowl. In wild ducks and wading birds, the Type A influenza viruses are normally avirulent, and cause no disease, suggesting that they are highly adapted to these species.

Swine influenza, the clinical disease in pigs, was first observed in 1918. Since then, it has increasingly been recognized that pigs are an important host for the influenza virus, as, unlike many other animal species, and because of the particular nature of the receptors for Type A influenza viruses that they bear on the cells of their respiratory tract, they are susceptible to direct infection with Type A strains originating from either humans or avian species, such infections arising because of the frequent and relatively consistent close contact of pigs with both humans and domestic poultry, particularly ducks and geese. Only haemagglutinin H1 and H3, and neuraminidase N1 and N2 antigens have so far been identified in pigs. The serotypes that are mainly responsible for disease, and are endemic in these animals, are H1N1 and H3N2; both of these Type A influenza serotypes are also present in humans. However, genetic sequence analysis suggests that there are two different genetic lineages of H1N1 strains present in pigs: one lineage comprises the classical H1N1 strains possibly derived initially from humans around 1918, while the other is most closely related to H1N1 strains initially isolated from ducks in the early 1980s, suggesting transmission from the latter into pigs around this time. The H3N2 serotype most commonly found in pigs is most closely related to the H3N2 influenza viruses circulating in humans during the 1970s, but more recently other H3N2 strains have been isolated from pigs in southern China, and genetic analysis of these strains suggests they may be derived from an avian source, probably ducks.

Unlike many mammals, the epithelial cells of the porcine respiratory tract carry receptors that can facilitate the attachment of both avian and human influenza viruses, thereby permitting viruses transmitted from either humans or avian species to enter and replicate in the cells of the pig. As a consequence of this, it is believed that the pig can act as a 'mixing vessel' allowing reassortment of the genes from such Type A avian and human influenza viruses in its respiratory tract, resulting in the formation of strains that may be novel for humans, therefore possessing pandemic potential.

Horses, donkeys, mules and other equidae can be infected by Type A influenza viruses, although only H7N7 and H3N8 have been reported in these animals since 1956. The H3N8 strain of virus was first isolated from horses in Miami in 1963. Many outbreaks of equine influenza occur in horse-racing stables or at racetracks, and such outbreaks have occasionally resulted in the suspension of horse-racing, leading to considerable economic loss. Over the winter of 1989–90, there was evidence of severe H3N8 infection in horses in north-eastern China, associated with a mortality rate of 20%. Genetic analysis of the virus responsible indicated it had spread recently into horses from an avian source, and was probably mutated from an avian influenza virus, suggesting that cross-species transmission from birds to horses had taken place. This virus was clearly distinguishable antigenically from the H3N8 strains already existing in horses in other parts of the world.

Various Type A influenza virus serotypes have been isolated from harbour seals, whales and domesticated mink. Genetic and antigenic analyses of these strains suggest that they have spread into these mammalian species from wild avian species, illustrating the regular cross-species transmission of the Type A influenza viruses. Occasional transmission from these species into humans coming into contact with these animals has been recorded.

Pathogenicity and virulence

Aquatic birds are reservoirs for all 15 HA subtypes of the Type A influenza viruses, and the cells lining the intestinal tract are the site of replication of these viruses in wild ducks. As avian serotypes of Type A influenza viruses cause no disease in wild birds, it is probable that, following transmission to a new host species (avian or otherwise), highly pathogenic strains of the virus can evolve from the normally avirulent serotypes in the wild bird host, and an important factor in this process are mutations in the highly mutable HA molecule affecting a site that is involved in the cleavage of this molecule that takes place in the early stages of viral replication. The presence of more than one basic amino acid at this cleavage site is associated with high levels of virulence in Type A avian influenza viruses. The H5 serotype of HA responsible for the lethality of the Type A influenza virus in chickens in 1997 may have originated from a strain of the virus known to be highly lethal in geese, A/Goose/Guangdong/1/96, and it is perhaps of some significance that the province of Guangdong in China is next to Hong Kong and supplies much of the latter's domestic poultry. Regardless of its origin, however, antigenic and genetic analysis indicates that the 2004–05 isolates of the H5N1 serotype are undergoing mutations close to the receptor-binding site of the virus, which will be affecting, through antigenic drift, both the antigenicity and receptor-binding specificity of the virus, and perhaps also its transmissibility. The HA antigens of Type A influenza viruses of avian origin attach to a sialic acid receptor of a particular specificity found on avian gut epithelial cells, but not on human respiratory tract epithelial cells. Consequently, such viruses cannot attach to and infect human respiratory tissue. Conversely, the receptor for human strains of Type A influenza virus present on human respiratory epithelial cells is not present on avian gut epithelium.

An important molecular factor that may be associated with the virulence of Type A influenza viruses and that may facilitate the invasion of many tissues, not merely the respiratory tract, in the avian, animal or human body following infection is the nature and availability of host endoproteases that are required to cleave the HA molecule of the virus. This cleavage is necessary to expose a fusogenic site at the amino terminus of one chain of the dimeric HA molecule that enables fusion to take place between the HA protein and the membrane of the intracellular vacuole that contains the virus particle after endocytosis. This fusion permits the viral replication cycle to continue. There is considerable evidence that Type A influenza viruses that are virulent in both domestic poultry and humans have their HA cleaved by intracellular endoproteases such as furin, while avirulent strains are dependent upon extracellular proteases such as plasmin or upon proteases from infecting or commensal bacteria, which are probably less readily available to them in the host tissues.

Although the surface HA and NA proteins are of major importance for the replication and virulence of Type A influenza viruses, it is becoming increasingly clear that some internal proteins of the virus may also contribute to the virulence and spread in the host. In particular, a single mutational substitution, of glutamic acid to lysine in the PB_2 protein of the polymerase enzyme complex of the virus, is believed to be of importance for adaptation from the avian to the mammalian host, probably increasing the replication efficiency of the virus in mammalian cells. Other mutations in genes coding for the polymerase complex of the virus – the PB_2 enzyme and the nucleocapsid protein (NP) gene segments – have also been identified in a laboratory-derived mutant virus that is highly lethal for mice.

Mutations in a further viral gene, that coding for the non-structural (NS_1) protein of the Type A influenza virus, may also play a role in increasing the pathogenicity of this virus for mammals – at least with respect to the H5N1 strains isolated in 1997. Strains of this virus having a single amino acid substitution in their NS_1 protein were found to have markedly increased resistance to the antiviral activity of interferon (IFN) and of tumour necrosis factor α (TNF-α) in cell culture, and also to induce severe disease in pigs.

Finally, it has been reported that patients infected with H5N1 strains of Type A influenza virus have considerably raised levels of an IFN-inducing chemokine, IP-10, present in their serum, and that H5N1 strains isolated in 1997 and 2004 are extremely potent at inducing this, and other chemokines and cytokines, in human primary alveolar and bronchial epithelial cells *in vitro*. These findings raise the possibility that cytokine dysregulation or imbalance may be a further factor contributing to the high pathogenicity of the H5N1 avian influenza viruses. Table 4.2 lists some of the factors that may contribute to the virulence of Type A influenza viruses.

However, all of the complex, and probably interacting, factors necessary to impart high

Table 4.2
Factors influencing the virulence of avian type A influenza viruses

Property	*Avirulent strains*	*Virulent strains*
Plaque formation in cell culture	Requires exogenous protease	No exogenous protease needed
HA cleavage	Cannot be achieved by intracellular proteases	Can be achieved by intracellular proteases
Sequence of HA cleavage site	Single arginine base	Multiple basic amino acids
Host enzymes eliciting cleavage of HA	Xa-like endoprotease *in ovo* Bacterial proteases (?) Endoprotease Clara (?)	Intracellular endoproteases, eg furin Plasmin endoprotease (?)
Phenotypic changes in the PB_2 protein	No	Yes (?)
Increased resistance to interferons and TNF-α	No	Yes (?)
Induction of pro-inflammatory cytokines	+	+++

HA, haemagglutinin; TNF-α, tumour necrosis factor α

pathogenicity and high virulence to Type A influenza viruses remain incompletely understood, although work with the avian strains suggest that broad tissue tropism and an ability to replicate rapidly in the host are major factors determining high pathogenicity in domestic chickens, and probably also in humans. The presence of a multibasic cleavage site in the HA molecule and mutation of a single specific amino acid in the PB2 internal protein of the virus appear to be of considerable importance. The highly pathogenic avian H5N1 viruses that have infected humans and the highly pathogenic H7N7 virus transmitted to humans in the Netherlands in 2003 both possess HA molecules with multiple basic amino acids at the cleavage site. In addition, the sole fatal human infection in the H7N7 Netherlands outbreak was caused by a virus possessing a mutated PB2 gene.

Clinical disease in the non-human host

Type A influenza infections in the non-human host can often be of considerable clinical, environmental and economic significance, and outbreaks of severe or lethal infections in domestic poultry, horses, pigs, cetaceans and, most recently, in dogs and felines, occur periodically.

In wild ducks, Type A influenza viruses cause no disease, although they can be excreted in high concentrations in the faeces. However, the transmission of such viruses into domestic chickens, ducks, geese and turkeys can produce a highly lethal disease spreading very rapidly in the local region and leading, in some of the recent outbreaks, to the loss of more than 100 million birds through the disease and culling. The first highly virulent outbreak of avian influenza in poultry was reported in 1959, and there have been 24 further outbreaks of this disease up to the present. Most of these outbreaks have not spread widely and have been confined to their area of origin. The symptoms of highly virulent Type A avian influenza virus infection in poultry, usually occurring after an incubation period ranging from 6 to 72 hours, are systemic in nature, involving the gut, as well as respiratory, reproductive and neurological organs, and include loss of appetite, cessation of egg laying, respiratory distress, diarrhoea, and discolouration of combs and wattles due to changes in blood circulation. In addition, sudden death can occasionally occur in the absence of any symptoms. In what may represent a significant development in the epidemiology of the H5N1 avian influenza viruses, it has recently been shown that domestic ducks can excrete this virus in their faeces in its lethal, highly virulent form, even though such birds remain healthy. This may therefore represent a route whereby virulent H5N1 Type A influenza strains may be silently transmitted to other poultry and, potentially, to humans. Such excretion has not been reported in ducks or other poultry in previous outbreaks of avian influenza.

Infection and illness in pigs is an acute respiratory one, and is in fact the commonest respiratory infection of these animals. Infection and disease usually occur through the introduction of pigs already infected with an influenza virus into a herd that has not previously experienced infection with that same strain or serotype, and that is therefore highly susceptible. Symptoms include fever, weight loss, coughing, nasal discharge and abortion. Most pigs will recover after a few days, but there may be complications of bronchopneumonia and secondary infections with other bacteria or viruses. Swine influenza can arise in an endemically infected herd annually, usually during the colder months of the year, and the virus is primarily spread from pig to pig via the nasopharyngeal route, with the virus being shed in nasal secretions, and disseminated through droplets or aerosols. It has been reported that the virus may be carried by some pigs for up to 3 months after their recovery.

Equine influenza, involving the H3N8 Type A influenza virus, is a disease of the upper respiratory tract, and illness can spread rapidly in racing stables, with fever, cough and nasal discharge. Transmission into a herd of horses or into a racing stable is usually through the introduction of a new animal into the existing group of animals. During the course of an outbreak, healthy adult horses that become infected normally recover in a week or so, provided that there are no secondary complications through bacterial infection, although sick animals can remain incapacitated for a few weeks and require a period of training to regain competitiveness.

In the outbreaks of H5N1 Type A avian influenza in felines (mainly tigers in zoos in Thailand), the infection has taken the form of a severe illness involving a serosanguinous nasal discharge and respiratory distress, high fever, increased levels of liver enzymes, neurological signs, leukopenia and thrombocytopenia. A number of deaths have occurred among the infected tigers.

Control

The mammalian and avian species that the Type A influenza viruses are known to infect, and the known and presumed transmission of these viruses between these species (and humans), are illustrated in Figure 4.1a. Also shown, (Figure 4.1b) are four control measures that can reduce the spread of these viruses between different species (and humans).

To control an outbreak of the highly virulent H5N1 Type A influenza virus in chickens and other domestic poultry, and especially to attempt to minimize the risk of the virus being transmitted to humans, it is necessary to cull all infected flocks, and any neighbouring flocks of birds liable to infection, accompanied by appropriate disposal of the carcasses. The complete cull in the poultry farms and the poultry markets in Hong Kong in December 1997 fully prevented any further spread of the H5N1 serotype to humans at that time. It is suggested that there should be some worldwide form of surveillance of avian and mammalian species for the detection of Type A influenza virus activity in various animal species that are of importance in the transmission of such viruses to humans. However, the experience with the spread of avian influenza to humans since 1997 suggests that such transmission may be difficult to contain, and it is even difficult

Relationships between avian, mammalian and human influenza viruses

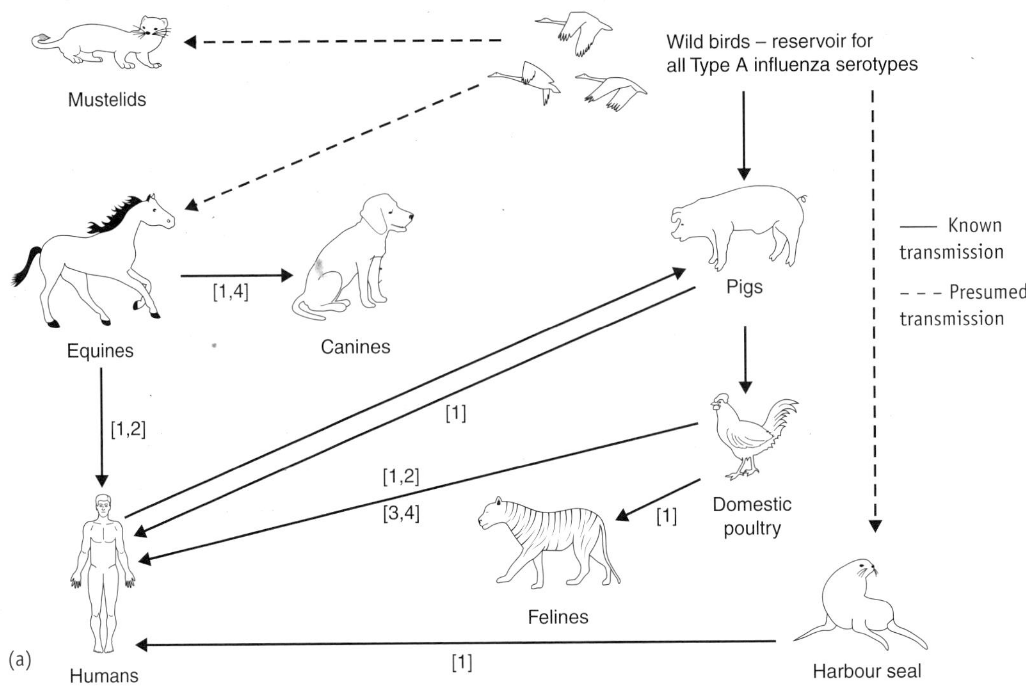

1. Avoid contact between species (eg housing poultry inside)

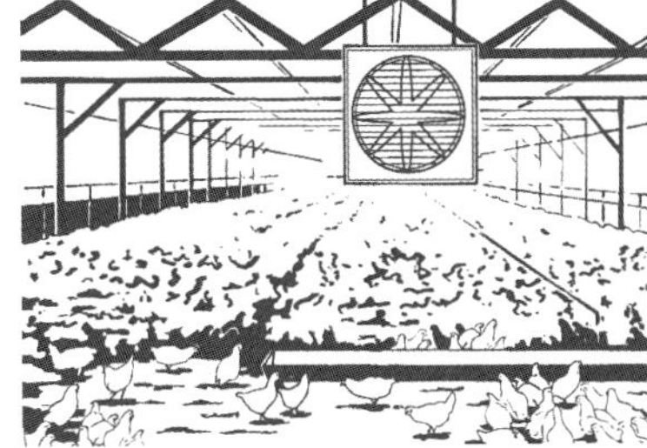

2. Culling the source animal species

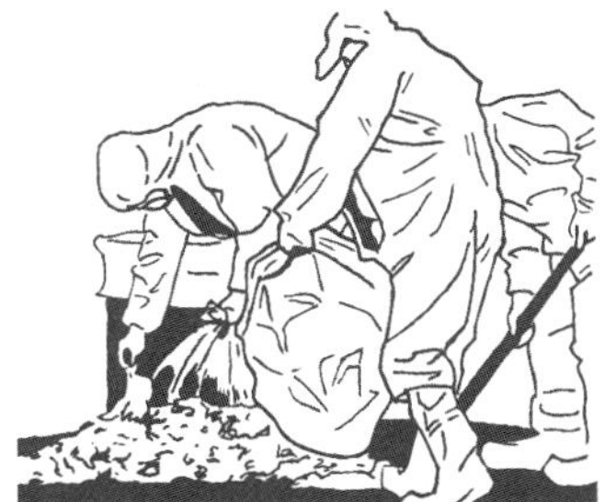

3. Immunization of the animal species

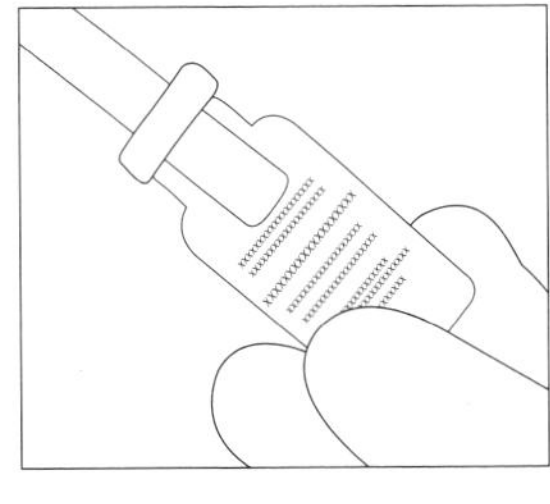

4. Preventing movement of the animal species (quarantine)

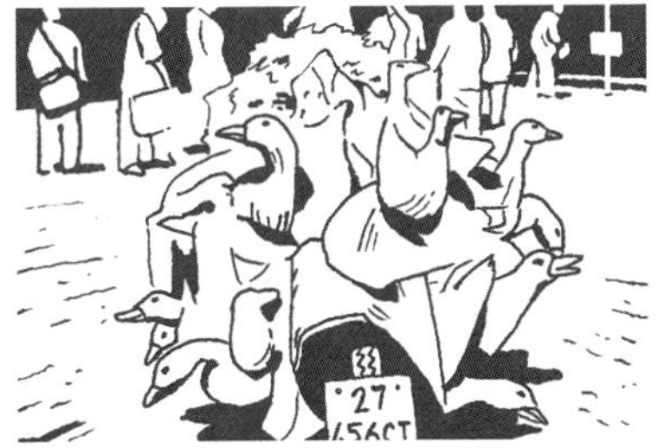

(b)

Figure 4.1
Influenza Type A transmitted between different animal species and humans (a); control measures that can reduce the spread of influenza Type A viruses between different animal species and humans (b).

to predict with certainty which of a number of avian strains may become adapted to, and transmitted between, humans, and have pandemic potential. Nevertheless, it is important to attempt to contain the H5N1 serotype, and other potentially highly virulent serotypes (particularly in birds) through early, sustained and aggressive culling policies. If these achieve a goal of limiting the number of events resulting in cross-species transmission to humans, this will reduce the number of opportunities the virus has for adaptation to the human host and the development of a virus with pandemic potential.

Other control measures may include the quarantining of infected poultry farms and the prevention of spread to neighbouring farms through contaminated cages, feed, clothing and other equipment, as during cold weather the virus can survive for long periods of time outside its host. If infection of a flock by a potentially lethal strain of Type A influenza is detected early enough, and the birds are culled, this may halt the infection before the virus is able to mutate and adapt to cause severe systemic and lethal disease in its new host. In 2005, a vaccine for use against H5N1 influenza virus strains in domestic poultry was developed, and has been used in some countries, notably China, but the efficacy of the vaccine and its success in preventing severe and lethal avian influenza infection in the poultry industry remains to be determined.

In pigs, the only effective way to control an outbreak of swine influenza is by complete depopulation, as, once established in a herd, the virus will persist, and spread into young animals and into any new, influenza-free, stock subsequently introduced into the herd.

Commercially prepared vaccines are available for use against influenza in horses and other equids; while not preventing infection, these can significantly reduce the severity of the clinical symptoms. Spread within a stable can be limited by isolating any newly acquired animals prior to introduction into the herd, and by the use of appropriate disinfectants.

Cross-species transmission

Transmission between non-human species

There is considerable transmission between different avian species, but of particular importance is the transmission between wild waterfowl, gulls and waders in general, and domesticated poultry (Figure 4.1). Such transmission is probably ongoing on a fairly regular basis. Two types of avian influenza infection are transmitted from wild waterfowl to farmed ducks, chickens, turkeys and geese – one that is common and mild, the second much rarer and highly lethal to the infected poultry. The Type A influenza viruses that can be of high pathogenicity for domestic poultry are particularly those subtypes bearing either the H5 or H7 antigen, but on initial infection of poultry these strains are avirulent, and it is only following spread within the infected flock and mutation of the viral genes providing adaptation to their host that they acquire virulence and lethality. In the past, by a similar process, Type A avian influenza viruses are believed to have spread to, and caused severe outbreaks of illness and disease, in pigs, horses, harbour seals and whales.

Transmission between mammals or birds and humans

Table 4.3 shows the numbers of cases and fatalities associated with the H5N1 influenza virus in humans, from January 2003 to June 2006. The H5 serotype was first reported as causing severe infection in humans in 1997.

New serotypes of Type A influenza viruses appearing in humans in 1957, 1968 and 1977 originated in China. The 1957 Asian pandemic was started by a virus (H2N2) that had acquired three new genes, coding for the HA and NA antigens and one internal protein, from an avian influenza virus by genetic reassortment, and these strains replaced the previously existing H1N1 strains, which disappeared completely from the human population. The Hong Kong pandemic of 1968 was caused by a virus that had acquired two

Table 4.3
Avian influenza cases and fatalities in humans 2003–June 2006

Country	Years	Cases	Deaths
Azerbaijan	2006	8	5
Cambodia	2005-06	6	6
China	2005-06	18	12
Djibouti	2006	1	0
Egypt	2006	14	6
Indonesia	2005-06	49	37
Iraq	2006	2	2
Thailand	2004-05	22	14
Turkey	2006	12	4
Vietnam	2003-05	93	42
Totals		225	128

new genes by reassortment – one coding for an internal viral protein, the other coding for the HA antigen. Both of these genes again originated from avian sources, probably from domestic ducks. This virus, an H3N2 serotype, retained the same gene coding for the NA antigen as was present in the preceding H2N2 strains. Following the H3N2 Hong Kong pandemic, the H2N2 serotype was no longer found in humans.

It is generally believed that, unlike the present situation, both the 1957 H2N2 and 1968 H3N2 serotypes of Type A influenza viruses did not spread directly from avian species into humans, but that the pig acted as an intermediate host or 'mixing vessel', and that both the H2N2 and H3N2 viruses arose by reassortment, in pigs, of Type A viral genes derived from an avian and a human virus, both of which happened to be infecting the pigs simultaneously. It has been established that pigs can be infected experimentally by all avian Type A serotypes (H1,...,H13) so far tested.

Prior to 1997, the H5 serotype of Type A influenza had never been reported in humans. Following the 1997 outbreak of the serotype H5N1 in Hong Kong, testing of faecal samples from ill chickens, ducks and geese demonstrated that virus was present in about 20% of the samples from chickens and in 2% of the samples from other domestic poultry. It became clear that the H5N1 virus was being spread to humans from the faeces of ill birds at the poultry markets in Hong Kong, and that both the virus and the disease were rife in birds on the poultry farms supplying the markets.

It is now well recognised that Type A influenza viruses can spread from pigs to humans and *vice versa*. Indeed, antigenically 'human-like' H3N2 strains are recognized in pigs, reflecting their origin in humans prior to their cross-transmission to these animals. As in humans, such strains may be subject to antigenic drift in the pig, although it is possible that some of the early H1N1 strains of the swine influenza virus have remained relatively unchanged in pig populations over a long period of time. Also, as in humans, Type A influenza viruses present in the pig may undergo genetic reassortment with other Type A influenza virus serotypes, derived from some avian species for example, that may infect, and therefore be present in the animal at the same time as the virus derived from human sources.

Further reading

Chan MCW, Cheung CY, Chui WH *et al.* Proinflammatory cytokine responses induced by influenza A (H5N1) viruses in primary human alveolar and bronchial epithelial cells. *Respir Res* 2005; **6**: 1–13.

Horimoto T, Kawaoka Y. Pandemic threat posed by avian influenza viruses. *Clin Microbiol Rev* 2001; **14**: 129–49.

Lipatov AS, Gororkova EA, Webby RJ *et al.* Influenza: emergence and control. *J Virol* 2004; **78**: 8951–9.

Seo SH, Hoffman E, Webster RG. Lethal H5N1 influenza viruses escape host anti-viral cytokine responses. *Nat Med* 2002; **8**: 950–4.

Webster R. The importance of animal influenza for human disease. *Vaccine* 2002; **20**: S16–20.

World Health Organization Global Influenza Program Surveillance Network. Evolution of H5N1 avian influenza viruses in Asia. *Emerging Infect Dis* 2005; **11**: 1515–21.

Writing Committee of the World Health Organization (WHO) Consultation on Human Influenza A/H5. Avian influenza A (H5N1) infection in humans. *N Engl J Med* 2005; **353**: 1374–85.

5. Clinical assessment

Symptoms in adults
Symptoms in children
Influenza virus pneumonia
Diagnosis
Influenza in pregnancy
Overview of management of seasonal influenza
Clinical features of avian influenza

Infection by Type A and B influenza viruses usually occurs in winter, with most outbreaks in the UK occurring during December–March. The incidence of 'influenza-like illness' (episodes where the patient is showing typical symptoms of influenza without confirmation by laboratory diagnosis) reported by general practitioners in the UK varies annually, but cases are seen in most years. In the UK, a weekly incidence of influenza-like illnesses greater than 400 per 100 000 of the population is considered to constitute an infection rate of epidemic proportions.

Symptoms in adults

Influenza caused by either Type A or B viruses is an acute infection with an incubation period of 2–3 days, and is a distinct clinical entity. Typically, the uncomplicated infection in adults is a tracheobronchitis with the additional involvement of the small airways. In addition to a high temperature (38–40°C), the patient normally suffers an abrupt onset of malaise, headache, chills and myalgia in the limbs and back, and will be confined to bed for a few days. A dry non-productive cough, occasionally accompanied by pharyngitis and nasal obstruction, may arise as the infection progresses.

Uncomplicated influenza in a healthy individual lasts from 3–7 days. The fever starts to decline approximately 3 days after the onset of symptoms. The patient's temperature is usually back to normal 5–6 days after onset. Although the physical findings are generally minimal, the patient can appear quite toxic, and a generalized weakness may persist in some individuals for a week or so after recovery from the major clinical signs and symptoms. Many patients with genuine influenza virus infection are so ill that they will voluntarily take to their beds and are reluctant to exert themselves. Influenza infection is normally more severe in cigarette smokers.

Although most influenza infections during an epidemic are clinically typical of influenza, a minority are either asymptomatic or manifest as simple rhinitis, sometimes accompanied by pharyngitis. The symptoms of uncomplicated influenza in adults and their duration are shown in Figure 5.1.

Symptoms in children

In children and younger individuals, influenza is generally of shorter duration, although the symptoms are essentially the same as in adults. There is a higher incidence of asymptomatic and minor infections in preschool and young schoolchildren than in adults. This is a factor associated with spread of the viruses by these cohorts of the population. Nevertheless, children can develop severe influenza infections, with high fever and occasionally febrile convulsions.

Symptoms that are seen more frequently in children than adults include:

- infections associated with the lower respiratory tract, such as croup and pneumonia
- extrapulmonary manifestations, such as vomiting, abdominal pain and myositis.

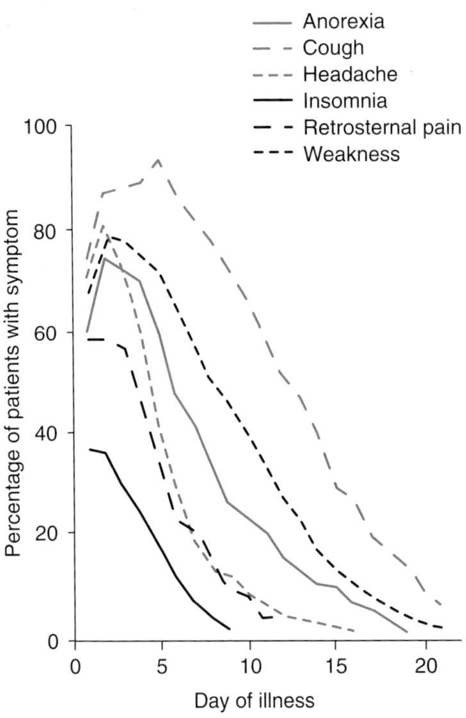

Figure 5.1
Frequency and duration of symptoms in 148 patients infected with the Type A/Hong Kong/68 influenza virus. [From Hobson *et al.* 1972.]

Myositis

Myositis is more commonly associated with Type B than with Type A influenza virus infection, and usually presents as the child is recovering from the illness. The first symptoms are acute pain and tenderness, particularly in the gastrocnemius and soleus muscles, resulting in extremely painful walking. Serum creatine phosphokinase levels are usually transiently elevated. Occasionally, myositis occurs as a result of direct viral invasion of the muscle, and the clinical symptoms are synchronous with the other, more usual, manifestations of influenza. Most patients recover completely after 3–4 days, although myoglobinuria and renal failure can sometimes occur. Very rarely, cardiac myositis occurs, with classic ECG changes of myositis, sometimes accompanied by tachydysrhythmias. Cardiac enzymes may be greatly elevated.

> The symptoms of influenza are essentially the same in children and adults, but last longer in adults

Reye's syndrome

Reye's syndrome is very occasionally associated with influenza virus infection in children, particularly during or following long-term aspirin therapy. The symptoms are consistent with acute encephalopathy with cerebral oedema. The patient usually has raised cerebrospinal fluid (CSF) pressure but normal CSF microscopy and biochemistry. This condition is associated with fatty degeneration of the liver, manifested as abnormal liver function tests and occasionally jaundice. However, this rare disease may be associated with other non-influenzal trigger factors.

Influenza virus pneumonia

Complications involving the lower respiratory tract can occur following influenza virus infection in both adults and children. These are usually seen in the groups particularly at risk from the infection, such as the elderly, in whom 80–90% of all influenza-related deaths occur. Individuals with chronic obstructive airways disease or other cardiopulmonary diseases are also at particular risk. Nevertheless, in the 1957 Asian influenza pandemic, when primary influenza virus pneumonia was first clearly documented, it was reported that one-quarter of these primary pneumonia cases occurred in normal, healthy individuals.

> Symptoms of influenza virus pneumonia include a rapid respiration rate, tachycardia, cyanosis, high fever and hypotension

Clinically, following the onset of influenza, a viral pneumonia accompanied by an overwhelming toxaemia characteristically develops within 24 hours. The symptoms include a rapid respiration rate, tachycardia, cyanosis, high fever and hypotension. Hypoxaemia and death may follow between 1 and 4 days later. Such severe and fatal infections are usually associated with Type A influenza viruses, but the pathogenesis of these toxaemic symptoms is not well understood. The virus replicates in and is confined to the epithelial cells of the respiratory tract. It is rarely detected in the blood of infected individuals. Under *in vitro* conditions, however, the virus can enter leukocytes, lymphocytes and macrophages, and may be able to exert certain biological effects, such as apoptosis, on these cells.

A chest X-ray of a patient with influenza virus pneumonia usually shows patchy consolidation in two or more lobes (Figure 5.2). Cavitation or pleural effusion implies bacterial superinfection. The pneumonia is an interstitial pneumonitis with severe hyperaemia and broadening of the alveolar walls, together with a mononuclear cell infiltration accompanied by capillary dilatation and thrombosis. This pathological presentation may also be produced by other viruses infecting the lower respiratory tract.

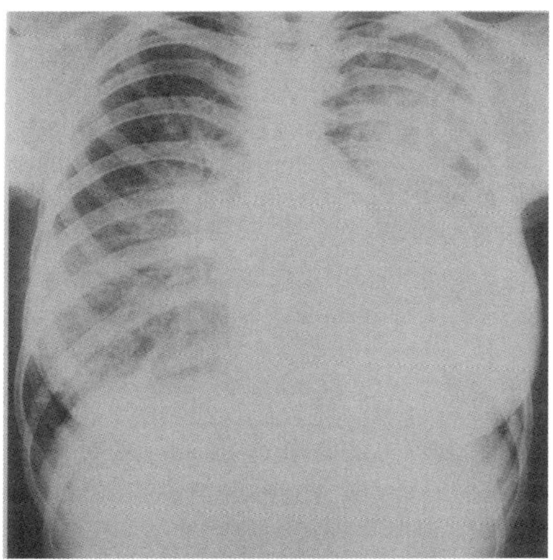

Figure 5.2
A typical X-ray presentation of fatal influenza virus pneumonia in an adult patient, showing acute lung congestion spread diffusely from the hilar region into the periphery and irregular soft mottling. [Reproduced from Mulder J, Hers JF. *Influenza*. Wolters Noordhoff, 1972.]

In influenza virus pneumonia, the virus replicates in the alveolar epithelial cells. Influenza-specific antigen can be detected in these cells and in alveolar macrophages. Initial improvement in those destined to survive occurs 5–16 days after onset of the pneumonia. In general, there are no lasting problems, although a minority of patients develop a diffuse interstitial fibrosis accompanied by impaired lung function.

During the major pandemic of 1957, a quarter of primary influenza virus pneumonia cases occurred in otherwise apparently healthy individuals

Diagnosis

Differential diagnosis of influenza is usually not possible on clinical grounds in non-epidemic periods, as the respiratory tract manifestations of the infection are common to those produced by other respiratory tract pathogens. During an influenza epidemic however, the disease is reasonably easy to diagnose clinically and without laboratory help. Moreover, during an epidemic attributable to Type A or B influenza, an adult with a diffuse interstitial pneumonia is likely to be suffering from influenza virus pneumonia.

A complete and reliable diagnosis of the infection can only be established with laboratory help:

- by recovery of the virus from clinical samples such as throat or nasal swabs or washings by culture
- by the detection of specific viral proteins or viral genetic material in such clinical specimens
- by the demonstration of increasing specific anti-influenza antibodies in serum or nasal washes.

Influenza in pregnancy

During the 2 or 3 years following the appearance of a novel pandemic influenza virus strain, there is an increased risk of women developing fatal influenzal disease during the second or third trimester of pregnancy. This increased risk was reported after both the 1918 and 1957 Type A influenza virus pandemics.

There is no definitive association of influenza virus infection with either congenital anomalies or haematological malignancies. The virus has only very rarely been isolated from either the maternal bloodstream or the fetus.

> After a novel virus pandemic, pregnant women are at risk of developing fatal influenzal disease

Overview of management of seasonal influenza

The management of influenza is based on the annual vaccination of those populations considered to be at the greatest risk either from infection by the viruses or from sequelae, such as secondary bacterial infections. Such groups include:

- those aged 65 years and above
- other groups who are immunocompromised for whatever reason
- those with chronic respiratory or heart disease
- diabetics.

See Chapter 7 for more detail on the use of influenza virus vaccines in the management of infection. Information on the ever-increasing numbers and use of anti-influenza drugs is given in Chapter 8.

Clinical features of avian influenza

Since 1997, there have been several small, yet severe, outbreaks of Type A influenza in humans in several parts of the world caused by viruses bearing non-human H5, H7 or H9 haemagglutinin antigens. These viruses have been transmitted to humans from domestic poultry sources, and the outbreaks have occurred despite the fact that avian Type A influenza viruses grow much less efficiently in human cells than in their natural avian host cells.

The clinical features of avian influenza differ from those of seasonal influenza, and all the outbreaks of human disease that have been described to date have arisen primarily in South East Asia and have followed association and intimate contact with birds. Among patients suffering disease due to H5N1 influenza, the prominent clinical features on admission to hospital were fever, cough, diarrhoea and shortness of breath. The incubation period following contact with birds has been calculated to be between 2 and 4 days. Some patients have developed pleuritic pain, and sputum is occasionally bloodstained. In contrast to seasonal influenza, sore throat, conjunctivitis and runny nose are not prominent symptoms. Physical examination generally reveals a fever, a rapid respiratory rate, respiratory distress and crackles on examination of the chest. The chest radiograph commonly shows widespread infiltrates.

Characteristic laboratory findings have included lymphopenia (depletion of $CD4^+$ T-helper lymphocytes in particular) and thrombocytopenia. Liver and renal dysfunction and hyperglycaemia have also been prominent laboratory features.

The two outbreaks that have been described in detail were from Vietnam and Hong Kong. In the Vietnam series, patients were generally young, but in the Hong Kong series, patients ranged up to 60 years of age. During the Hong Kong outbreak of 1997, of 18 people with confirmed infection, 6 died. Many of these patients suffered from:

- severe haemorrhagic complications
- renal failure.

Following mass culling of poultry and other successful infection control measures, no new cases were detected until February 2003, when two cases were reported, one of whom died. In the Thai outbreak of 2004, 8 of 10 patients died. In this outbreak, all patients were treated empirically with broad-spectrum antibiotics, and 7 of the 10 patients received methylprednisolone. Five patients were treated with oseltamivir and one received oseltamivir with ribavirin. The median time to death from onset of the illness was 9 days.

The severity of this infection in apparently healthy individuals aged 13–60 years has been of considerable concern, creating a new awareness of the direct infective potential of avian influenza viruses for humans. Nevertheless, this virus did not spread from one patient to another at this time, and did not therefore become established in humans.

The World Health Organization has been monitoring cases of avian influenza in humans, and up to June 2006, a total of 225 human cases were reported from nine countries between January 2004 and June 2006. Most cases were reported from Vietnam, Indonesia and Thailand and 128 people have died from the disease. Most avian influenza virus infections have been due to direct exposure to poultry, but there have been scattered reports of person-to-person transmission as evidenced by molecular epidemiology and the absence of exposure to birds.

Further reading

Hien TT, Liem NT, Dung NT *et al* Avian influenza A (H5N1) in 10 patients in Vietnam. *N Engl J Med* 2004; **350**: 1179–88.

Hobson D, Beare AS, Ward-Gardner A. Haemagglutination-inhibiting serum antibody titres as an index of the response of volunteers to intranasal infection with live attenuated strains of influenza virus. In: *Proceedings of Symposium on Live Influenza Vaccines*. Zagreb: Yugoslav Academy of Sciences and Arts, 1972: 73–84.

Murphy BR, Webster RG. Orthomyxoviruses. In: Fields BN, Knipe DM, Chanock RM *et al* (eds). *Fields' Virology*, 3rd edn, Vol 1. Philadelphia: Raven Press, 1990: 1091–152.

Oliviera EC, Marik PE, Colice G. Influenza pneumonia: a descriptive study. *Chest* 2001; **119**: 1717.

Ungchusak K, Auewarakul P, Dowell SF *et al.* Probable person-to person transmission of avian influenza A H5N1. *N Engl J Med* 2005; **352**: 333–40.

Yuen KY, Chan PK, Peiris M *et al.* Clinical features and rapid diagnosis of human disease associated with avian influenza A (H5N1) virus. *Lancet* 1998; **351**: 467–71.

6. Complications and 'at-risk' populations

The immunocompromised patient
Secondary bacterial complications
Conclusions

Severe and frequently fatal complications are caused by secondary bacterial infections in certain 'at-risk' groups of the population. These groups include:

- the elderly or debilitated, particularly those aged 75 years and above
- persons with chronic respiratory disease, including asthmatics and chronic bronchitics
- diabetics
- individuals with chronic and ischaemic heart disease
- immunocompromised individuals
- individuals with renal disease
- residents of closed institutions, where attack rates during an influenza epidemic may be extremely high.

> If associated with Type A influenza viruses, secondary bacterial infections can be particularly harmful

In persons over 65 years with two or more high-risk conditions for influenza, the death rate attributable to influenza is 0.8%, compared with 0.02% in those aged 45–64 with no chronic disease conditions. In the over-65 age group, people at the highest risk of contracting influenza are those who have cardiovascular disease in combination with either chronic obstructive pulmonary disease (COPD) or diabetes mellitus.

The immunocompromised patient

All individuals in the 'at-risk' groups of the population will be compromised to some degree with respect to one or more elements of their non-specific or specific immune defences. This situation may arise through:

- the natural course of events (for example, there is a decline in immune response with advancing years, due to involution of the thymus gland: this is a process that results in a reduction in the functioning mass of the gland, producing a T-cell insufficiency)
- a decrease in T-lymphocyte function in the elderly, resulting in a drop in both the quality and quantity of the T-cell help delivered to other components of the immune system, including B cells.

These factors, together with the elimination of lymphocytes of various specificities throughout adult life, result in a characteristically changed immunological repertoire in the elderly. In some people, an immunocompromised state or an inadequately functioning respiratory tract may have been acquired through occupational disease or excessive smoking.

The number of young people at risk of death during an influenza virus epidemic or pandemic has increased due to the increased survival rates of:

- children with congenital diseases (eg cystic fibrosis and inherited immunodeficiencies)
- organ transplant patients
- HIV patients.

Secondary bacterial complications

Each year, many thousands of deaths are attributable to secondary bacterial diseases following an influenza virus infection. The bacteria most frequently involved are *Streptococcus pneumoniae*, *Staphylococcus aureus* and *Haemophilus influenzae*. Infection with *S. aureus* affects the lung by causing oedema, hyperaemia, haemorrhaging, consolidation and formation of pus (Figure 6.1).

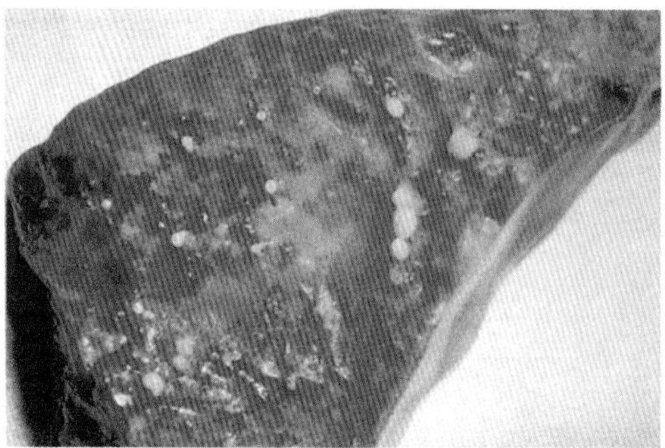

Figure 6.1
Gross appearance at postmortem of the lung following *Staphylococcus aureus* infection secondary to influenza virus infection, showing oedema, hyperaemia, haemorrhaging, consolidation and the presence of pus.
[Reproduced from Mulder J, Hers JF. *Influenza*. Wolters Noordhoff, 1972.]

Pathogenesis

Interestingly, although influenza viruses preferentially replicate in the epithelial cells of the upper respiratory tract, they can also grow in leukocytes and peripheral blood monocytes. The viruses are able – at least under laboratory conditions – to induce apoptosis (programmed cell death) in these cells through the activity of the non-structural protein NS_1. Infection of humans with Type A influenza viruses has been reported to cause a severe but transient leukopenia. In recent experimental infections, some volunteers (around 10%) developed severe T-cell lymphopenia and moderate B-cell lymphopenia. However, 90% of these volunteers showed normal serum antibody responses. During the inflammatory processes associated with both uncomplicated influenza virus infection and secondary bacterial infections, leukocytes are recruited into the airways. Apoptosis of these cells is triggered by the infecting virus and could play a role in pathogenesis. This programmed cell death allows increased bacterial growth and multiplication because the efficiency of a major bacterial defence mechanism – the uptake and destruction of bacteria by leukocyte – is reduced.

Morbidity

In the UK, deaths from secondary bacterial infection subsequent to influenza virus infection are reflected in the figures of excess mortality, derived from the annually published national mortality statistics. The figures of excess mortality represent the number of deaths actually observed above the number of expected deaths over a given time period. In a winter period showing epidemic activity of a Type A influenza virus, the excess mortality figures are considerably higher than in a non-epidemic winter. This is almost entirely due to deaths (mainly in the elderly) from secondary bacterial pneumonia following influenza virus infection. Table 6.1 shows the excess deaths in England and Wales for all age groups of the population over 10 winters spanning the time period from 1989/90 through to 1998/99. The table indicates that most deaths were seen in the winters of 1989/90 and 1996/97.

Over the winter of 1994/95, there were fewer observed deaths than were expected, although this was a period of prolonged Type B influenza activity (Table 6.1). This indicates the lower virulence of this virus compared with Type A. Furthermore, the H3N2 subtype of the Type A virus was active during all but three of these winters, with Type B influenza being the active virus in 1990/91 and 1992/93 as well as in 1994/95. There was no significant outbreak associated with the H1N1 Type A influenza subtype over this period, suggesting either a greater degree of immunity to this virus in the general population or a lower intrinsic H1N1 virus virulence, or a combination of both factors.

Annual data on the excess number of people presenting with influenza-like illness (over the baseline rate of incidence) are issued from the Royal College of General Practitioners (RCGP). These excess numbers of consultations, for all age groups of the population, are also shown in Table 6.1. During 1989–99, an average of 421 872 individuals per year sought consultations for influenza-like illnesses.

Table 6.1
Excess deaths and estimates of excess consultations for influenza-like illness in England and Wales over 10 influenza seasons

Influenza season	*Influenza virus type/subtype active*	*Duration of epidemic (weeks)*	*Excess deaths in all age groups*	*Excess consultations for influenza-like illness in all age groups*
1989/90	H3N2	10	25 202	831 621
1990/91	B	12	11 356	276 064
1991/92	H3N2	11	6 707	266 525
1992/93	B	9	4 358	213 820
1993/94	H3N2	10	16 455	578 427
1994/95	B	14	−1 562	357 460
1995/96	H3N2	11	15 199	430 887
1996/97	H3N2	13	27 587	782 190
1997/98	H3N2	9	4 873	130 858
1998/99	H3N2	9	15 369	350 872
Mean	–	–	12 554	421 872

Adapted from Goddard NL, Joseph CA, Zambon M *et al.* Influenza surveillance in England and Wales: October 1999 to May 2000. *Commun Dis Public Health* 2000; **3**: 261–6. With kind permission of the PHLS Communicable Disease Surveillance Centre ©PHLS.

Clinical features

There are certain conditions that act as significant risk factors when sufferers contract influenza. Scientists are gradually beginning to understand the underlying factors that may precipitate serious or even fatal illness in these individuals. The common theme is the immunocompromised state, but this has many differing facets, which may be manifest in a variety of ways.

Chronic obstructive pulmonary disease

In COPD, excessive smoking, environmental pollution and prior infections may cause inflammatory damage to conducting airways and impair mucociliary clearance. This can lead to bacterial superinfection of the respiratory tract by, for example, *H. influenzae*, *Moraxella catarrhalis* and *S. pneumoniae*. Indeed, the patient is often colonized by these bacteria. Exacerbations associated with COPD include shortness of breath, cough and sputum production. Infection by Type A and B influenza viruses can lead to serious lower respiratory tract episodes involving one or more of the above-mentioned species.

Bronchiectasis

Bronchiectasis is a chronic condition of the respiratory tract. In bronchiectasis, as in COPD, the bronchial tree is heavily colonized by bacteria, and the patient suffers a chronic cough, haemoptysis, copious sputum production and general ill health. The disease is usually the result of a severe bacterial respiratory tract infection, such as whooping cough or pulmonary tuberculosis. It presents as an irreversible and abnormal dilatation of the bronchi with chronic inflammatory and fibrotic changes.

Cystic fibrosis

Cystic fibrosis is a genetically inherited autosomal recessive disease. The respiratory tract of affected neonates, infants and children is colonized by bacteria such as *S. aureus* and *H. influenzae*. In patients with advanced disease, various species of mucoid and non-mucoid pseudomonads also cause colonization. The viscous respiratory tract secretions in patients with cystic fibrosis tend to block the small airways, producing bronchiectasis.

> Patients with a compromised respiratory tract who contract influenza have an increased risk of severe or fatal bacterial overgrowth and invasion of the lungs

Ischaemic heart disease

The deaths occurring in individuals with ischaemic heart disease during an influenza epidemic may be explained by:

- the increased myocardial demands associated with the fever and hypoxia caused by viral infection
- the viral myocarditis that can sometimes occur in influenza virus infection.

In addition, the inflammatory response accompanying the infection may create a prothrombotic state, leading to an acute thrombotic cardiovascular event.

HIV

HIV infection impairs cellular immune responses, and humoral immunity is also affected. Resistance to infection by the influenza virus is primarily achieved through the presence of antibodies to the viral surface proteins at the time of infection. Recovery from the disease is mediated partly by cellular immune mechanisms – principally through the action of cytotoxic T lymphocytes. Thus, individuals with HIV infection or with acquired immunodeficiency syndrome (AIDS) will be at particular risk during an influenza epidemic.

Diabetes

Individuals over 65 years of age with diabetes mellitus who contract influenza have a six fold increased risk of hospitalization, and the mortality in such hospitalized persons is relatively high. The risk from influenza virus infection in this group appears to be related to the cardiovascular complications of diabetes rather than to the diabetes itself. Infection with the influenza virus, or the complications associated with the infection, may, however, cause a loss of metabolic control in diabetic patients. This results in an increase in glycosylated serum proteins and in ketoacidosis. Therefore, the hospitalization rate increases, as do the incidence of long-term complications and the mortality rate.

Asthma

In children suffering from asthma, influenza virus infection leads to exacerbations of wheezing and increased risk of hospitalization. It has been estimated that 24–85% of all asthma attacks in children are associated with viral respiratory tract infections – respiratory syncytial virus (RSV) infection is the most common, but influenza can also aggravate asthma.

Smoking

Smoking has not been reported to be a significant risk factor for hospitalizations or fatalities, despite the fact that it has been reported to be a risk factor for contracting influenza virus infection both in healthy young men and in a general population with a mean age of 44 years. However, infections are said to be more severe in cigarette smokers. Smoking does not appear to be a special risk factor for the elderly.

> Smoking has been reported as a risk factor for contracting influenza virus infection, but not for hospitalizations or fatalities

Conclusions

Influenza continues to have a considerable impact on the health of the nation. There is a potentially severe or fatal outcome in the significant and increasing proportion of the population that is already at some degree of risk due to age and/or chronic ill health. This is so, despite the availability since the 1970s of a vaccine known to be both safe and (at least where there is concordance between the infecting virus and the viral antigens present in the vaccine) effective. The problem of influenza thus resides in the peculiar properties of the virus itself. It remains a continuing challenge to find a novel vaccine or means of immunization, or to discover a novel drug that can successfully overcome – or at the very least markedly diminish – the frequent and regular effects of this virus on human communities around the world.

Further reading

Couch RB. Influenza: prospects for control. *Ann Intern Med* 2000; **133**: 992–8.

Cruijff M, Thijs C, Govaert T *et al.* The effect of smoking on infuenza, influenza vaccination efficacy and on the antibody response to influenza vaccination. *Vaccine* 1999; **17**: 426–32.

Das P. Flu experts feel countries are unprepared for a future pandemic. Lancet 2001; **357**: 1419.

Kramarz P, DeStefano F, Garguillo PM *et al.* Influenza vaccination in children with asthma in health maintenance organizations. Vaccine Safety Datalink Team. *Vaccine* 2000; **18**: 2288–94.

Nichols JE, Niles JA, Roberts NJ Jr. Human lymphocyte apoptosis after exposure to influenza A virus. *Virology* 2001; **73**: 5921–9.

Nicholson KG. Impact of influenza and respiratory syncytial virus on mortality in England and Wales from January 1975 to December 1990. *Epidemiol Infect* 1996; **116**: 51–63.

Simonsen L, Clarke MJ, Schonberger LB *et al.* Pandemic versus epidemic influenza mortality: a pattern of changing age distribution. *J Infect Dis* 1998; **178**: 53–60.

Webster RG. Immunity to influenza in the elderly. *Vaccine* 2000; **18**: 1686–9

7. Immunization

Efficacy
Groups recommended for vaccination
Vaccine production
Safety
Problems
Determination of vaccine immunogenicity
New strategies of vaccination
Local and systemic immune mechanisms
Novel vaccines
Use of vaccines in general practice

The first vaccines against influenza, developed and used in the 1950s and 1960s, consisted simply of complete virus particles killed by treatment with formaldehyde. These vaccines were relatively crude and impure, and were liable to give rise to both cutaneous reactions at the injection site and systemic side-effects, particularly fever, in an unacceptable proportion of the recipients. Although such vaccines, albeit in a much more highly purified form, remain available today, the influenza virus vaccines currently in use in the UK contain only the surface haemagglutinin (HA) and neuraminidase (NA) glycoproteins of the virus (Figure 7.1). These non-living protein preparations are thus extremely pure and are well tolerated by recipients following intramuscular injection. They are the only form of influenza virus vaccine recommended for children under 12 years of age, as killed whole virus vaccines may elicit systemic reactions, including high fever, in this age group.

> Surface antigen vaccines are the only form of influenza virus vaccine recommended for children under 12 years of age

Efficacy

Although their record on safety in all age groups of the population is excellent, surface antigen influenza virus vaccines do not demonstrate the very highest degree of efficacy (in terms of neither the humoral and cell-mediated immune responses that they induce, nor the protection rates that they achieve). This is especially true when there is a lack of close concordance between the viral antigens present in the vaccine and the viral strains circulating and causing infection in the general population. Even when close concordance does exist, there is often a lowered vaccine efficacy because of underlying problems relating to poor immune responses in recipients of the vaccine. These decreased immune responses may be due to:

- immune senescence in the elderly
- an immune system compromised through infections with viruses such as HIV or treatments with immunosuppressive drugs as in cancer or organ transplant patients.

Patients in these groups are at increased risk of severe or even fatal illness during an influenza virus epidemic. Hence, these groups are among the primary targets for influenza vaccination. It is clear that improvements in the nature of the vaccine or in the mode of its administration to the patient are necessary in order to provide adequate protection through the regularly occurring influenza virus epidemics.

> Primary targets for influenza vaccination are patients with compromised immune systems

Groups recommended for vaccination

Table 7.1 lists those groups for whom influenza vaccination is currently recommended in the

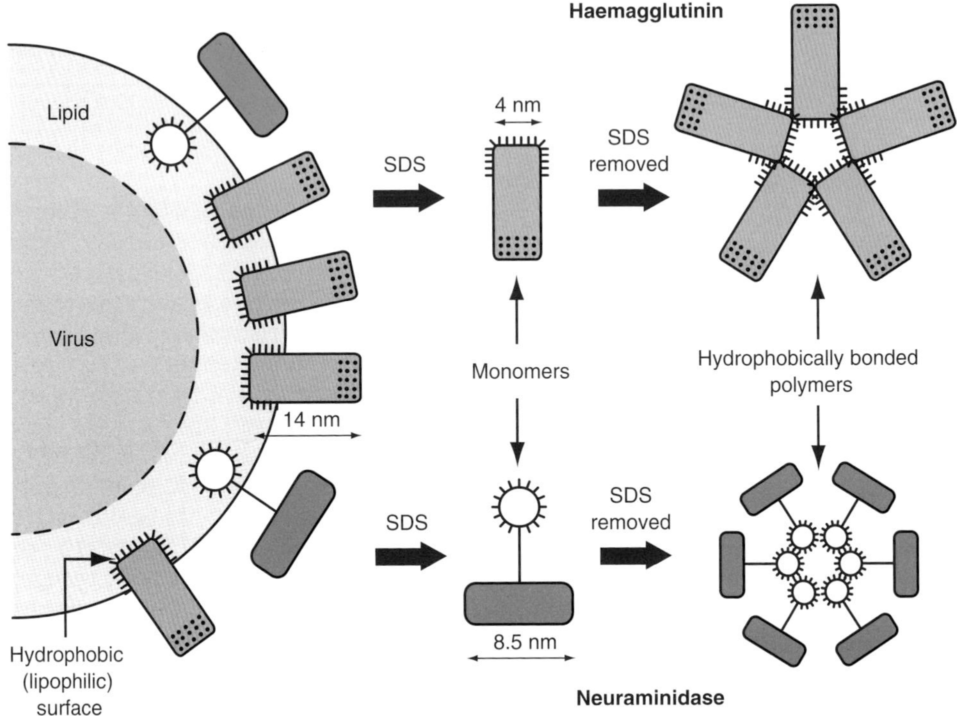

Figure 7.1
Schematic diagram showing the principles employed in the preparation of a surface antigen influenza vaccine. (SDS, sodium dodecyl sulfate.) [Adapted from Laver WG, Valentine RC. Morphology of the isolated haemagglutinin and neuraminidase subunits of influenza virus. *Virology* 1969; **38**: 105–19. With kind permission from Academic Press, Orlando, FL.]

UK. In addition, it is recommended that immunization be offered to all healthcare workers involved in the delivery of patient care and support. It is particularly important that these groups have some protection during an influenza epidemic, as the reduction in such support at these times may impose major strains on the capacity of the health services to deal with the epidemic. This can then lead to the development of an emergency situation.

Although vaccination is not recommended for healthy children or for adults under the age of 65, infection in these groups may still lead to an economic burden in terms of the number of working days and schooldays lost during even a mild influenza outbreak.

> It is recommended that immunization be offered to all healthcare workers involved in the delivery of patient care and support

Vaccine production

Influenza virus vaccines are currently manufactured in embryonated hen's eggs. The H3N2 and H1N1 Type A and the Type B influenza virus strains whose surface HA and NA proteins are to be incorporated in the vaccine for Europe are selected by the World Health Organization (WHO) in March each year. This selection is based on information obtained through the Influenza Surveillance Network, which involves over 100 laboratories around the

Table 7.1
Groups recommended for annual vaccination against influenza

- All persons aged over 65 years
- Individuals of all ages with chronic respiratory disease:
  - chronic obstructive pulmonary disease
  - bronchiectasis
  - asthma
  - cystic fibrosis
- Individuals of all ages with chronic cardiac disease
- Individuals of all ages with chronic renal disease
- Individuals with diabetes mellitus
- Immunosuppressed individuals:
  - leukaemias and other cancers
  - organ transplant patients
  - HIV/AIDS patients
- Individuals in long-stay residential accommodation

world that report to four WHO collaborating centres. The Influenza Surveillance Network monitors and reports on the incidence and severity of influenza outbreaks worldwide. It focuses particularly on the strains of virus causing these epidemics, including any changes seen in the surface proteins. Any detectable change in the antigenic nature of the surface proteins (particularly HA) of a newly isolated strain of influenza virus, which may indicate the possible development of a widespread outbreak or epidemic of influenza, will result in a recommendation to the vaccine manufacturers that these antigens be included in the vaccine for use in the following winter. The European manufacturers then have from April to October to prepare a sufficient amount of the recommended vaccine formulation.

Preparation of the vaccine commences with propagation of the recommended virus strains in a licensed cell system – usually well-characterized and pathogen-free embryonated hen's eggs.

The licensed cell culture system is also inoculated simultaneously, in order to obtain dually infected cells, using well-categorized, laboratory-adapted and genetically stable strains of either H3N2 virus (simultaneously with the current, recommended H3N2 virus) or H1N1 virus (simultaneously with the current, recommended H1N1 virus). These stable, laboratory-adapted 'master' strains of H3N2 and H1N1 are of low or no virulence for humans, but are capable of growing rapidly and to high levels in embryonated hen's eggs, the licensed cell culture system. The intention is to engineer a dual infection in the eggs such that both the current and laboratory-adapted H3N2 (or H1N1) strains can undergo genetic reassortment. This enables the production of progeny reassortant viruses that carry genes and bear the surface protein antigens of the currently circulating H3N2 or H1N1 strains, while at the same time possessing genes coding for viral internal proteins that are derived from the respective 'master' strains and confer on the reassortants the phenotypic characteristics of:

- rapid and high-yield growth characteristics in eggs
- a high degree of characterization and genetic stability with respect to their internal proteins
- the surface HA and NA proteins of the currently circulating, recommended strains required in the vaccine

> Influenza virus vaccines are produced in a licensed cell system, which is usually well-characterized, pathogen-free embryonated hen's eggs

Subsequent growth of these reassortants produces large quantities of virus bearing the required surface proteins. These are removed from the virus, normally through the use of surface-active agents, and purified for use in the vaccine.

Reassortment techniques are not used for the Type B influenza component of the vaccine. However, surface HA and NA proteins from the current circulating Type B virus are used in the vaccine following:

- cultivation of the virus in embryonated eggs
- separate the surface proteins using surface-active agents
- purification of the surface proteins.

The difficulties associated with influenza vaccine technology include poor growth of current virus strains in eggs and problems in obtaining the required reassorted virus at the reassortment stage. Both of these problems can prolong the time taken for vaccine production, delay the availability of vaccine for widespread use and affect the quantities of vaccine that can readily be prepared. The safety factors inherent in these procedures (especially the elimination of any potential virulence factors associated with the internal proteins of the cirulating wild-type viruses) are important, although in the face of an impending influenza pandemic caused by a strain of virus that is new to humans, large quantities of an effective, rapidly available vaccine will be needed urgently.

In recent years, a number of the major pharmaceutical companines have been researching and developing novel influenza vaccines using cell culture systems as a substrate for propagation of the virus rather than the embryonated hen's egg. Although such culture systems have some advantages over eggs for influenza virus growth, for example permitting a more appropiate structure for the surface HA protein antigen of the virus, there are concerns that it may be harder to achieve rapid, large-scale production of influenza vaccine in these cell culture systems.

Safety

The current surface protein influenza virus vaccines are very safe. They consist of the HA and NA antigens from the two Type A virus strains together with the HA and NA antigens from a single Type B influenza virus. In several studies in healthy adults, at dosage levels four times that currently used, these vaccines have been found to induce systemic reactions (such as raised temperature) no more frequently than in individuals receiving a placebo preparation.

These surface protein influenza virus vaccines are also safe in children under 2 years of age. Furthermore, there is no evidence of raised temperatures or febrile convulsions in this age cohort. These side-effects have been reported for the killed whole-virus vaccines, but such preparations are not available for use in the UK.

Most studies have reported a low level, (about 5%), of local reactions at the injection site following administration of the commercially available surface protein influenza virus vaccines. These reactions are mild and transient, lasting only 24–48 hours. Local or systemic allergic reactions to the highly purified surface protein influenza virus vaccines are very uncommon. Most of the reactions probably occur in people with egg allergies and are precipitated by the minute amount of egg protein that is residual in the vaccine. The use of the current egg-grown vaccines is contraindicated in individuals with egg allergies.

Exceptionally rarely, immunization against influenza has also been associated with Guillain–Barré syndrome.

> Vaccination is contraindicated in individuals with egg allergies

Problems

The limitations in efficacy of the current influenza virus vaccines have been mentioned earlier and are mainly due to two factors.

First, it has not proved possible to predict correctly the exact antigenic nature of the strains of virus that will be circulating during a forthcoming influenza season. Despite considerable theoretical and experimental work aimed at defining the nature of the mutations that take place in the viral genome, and searching for trends in past mutations in the genes coding for the surface proteins through the construction of phylogenetic trees, it is still impossible to anticipate these changes with any degree of accuracy. Therefore, in any given influenza epidemic, there will be a less than perfect match between the vaccine antigens and the circulating virus strains.

Second, the prime target groups at whom the vaccine is aimed – the elderly and the chronically ill – are often less than fully competent in their immune responses. The protection rates achieved following vaccination of these groups may be much lower than those elicited by the same vaccine in a healthy population. Some studies have reported protection rates as low as 20% in the elderly following immunization with a vaccine that matched the circulating influenza virus strains. Healthy young adults receiving the same vaccine under similar circumstances had a protection rate of 70%.

Determination of vaccine immunogenicity

The immunogenicity of current commercially available and novel experimental influenza virus vaccines is primarily assessed by determination of the levels of antibodies to the surface proteins of the virus (particularly the HA antigen) circulating in the blood of vaccine recipients. The level of such serum antibody that can be equated with a 50% chance of protection against infection by an influenza virus has been determined. European guidelines for the registration of influenza virus vaccines recommend that new, experimental influenza vaccines should elicit such protective levels of antibody in 75% of vaccine recipients.

New strategies of vaccination

Since the current commercially available influenza vaccines do not always provide a high level of protection, there is considerable interest in the further improvement of these vaccines either:

- through modification of the vaccines themselves, or
- through the way in which they are delivered.

Natural infection by the influenza viruses is acquired via the respiratory tract, with the virus initiating its replication in the lining mucosal epithelial cells. Both the virological and the host defence factors (specific and non-specific) associated with the initiation and progress of the infection are presented in Table 7.2.

Table 7.2
Events associated with establishment of influenza virus infection in the respiratory tract

Viral event	*Non-specific host defence effector mechanisms operating*	*Specific immune host defence mechanisms that will operate if present*
Initial presence at mucosal surface	Mucus viscosity Mucociliary escalator Proteases present in local secretions	Nil
Attachment and entry into susceptible cells	Mucus viscosity Mucociliary escalator Proteases in secretions	Locally produced IgA IgG transudated from the circulation
Replication inside susceptible cells	Interferon Apoptosis (programmed cell death)?	Nil
Presence and release of virus from infected cell surface	Natural killer cells	Cytotoxic T lymphocytes Locally produced IgA IgG transudated from the circulation
Extracellular spread of virus in the respiratory tract	Complement	Locally produced IgA IgG transudated from the circulation

IgA/G, immunoglobulin A/G

It is unlikely that an influenza vaccine given by injection into the deltoid muscle of the upper arm will induce appropriate antibody levels in the secretions bathing either the upper or the lower respiratory tract in the days and weeks following immunization. It is also unlikely that such antibody levels will be sustained over a whole influenza season. It is for these reasons that novel vaccines are under investigation.

Local and systemic immune mechanisms

The major antibody isotype present in mucosal secretions throughout the body is immunoglobulin A (IgA). This is produced locally at the mucosal surfaces and is relatively short-lived. The longer-lasting IgG antibody isotype, which is the major isotype produced in response to parenteral antigenic stimulation, forms only a minor component of respiratory tract secretions. It is believed to enter these secretions by transudation from the blood vessels underlying the respiratory mucosa. This transudation is greatest when there is some degree of inflammation in the respiratory tract. Inflammation can be brought about by, for example, infection with bacteria or viruses, including influenza. Ideally, to prevent infection of the respiratory tract mucosa by an invading influenza virus, the presence and immediate secretion of locally produced IgA is an important prerequisite. The presence of such antibody in the secretions bathing the respiratory mucosal surfaces at the time of infection can prevent attachment of the virus to susceptible host cells. If supported by non-specific host defences, such as natural killer cells and interferon destroying those cells that do become invaded by the virus, IgA should provide protection against the establishment of infection and development of the clinical symptoms of influenza. The closeness of the match between the anti-HA IgA antibodies and the HA protein present on the surface of the invading virus is also of considerable relevance here.

Intramuscular injection of the current influenza vaccines can promote high levels of durable systemic IgG and also memory cells that are able to respond in the event of subsequent infection. However, there will be a delay before these effector mechanisms are translated to, and are operating at, the respiratory mucosal surfaces. The immune actions of IgG and memory cells may not be transudated to the respiratory secretions until the inflammatory effects resulting from the infection are well under way and the virus is established in the respiratory tract tissues. Therefore, a major role for these specific defence mechanisms may be in limiting the spread of the virus and clearing an influenza virus infection that is already established in the respiratory tract.

Delivery by the nasal route

Because of the relevance of local specific immune mechanisms, particularly the activity of secretory IgA, in the prevention of influenza virus infection at the respiratory tract mucosal surfaces, the administration of an influenza vaccine via the nasal route (probably by means of a spray mechanism) is currently receiving considerable attention. If delivery of a surface protein influenza vaccine by this route can achieve high levels of local IgA in nasal secretions, and if these levels can be sustained over the entire influenza season (perhaps through periodic 'top-up' intranasal spray inoculations), then an important component of the specific defences required to prevent the initiation and establishment of infection by the virus will have been implemented. This is probably not a feature of the current intramuscularly injected vaccines.

Direct vaccine delivery by a nasal spray could achieve high levels of IgA antibody in nasal secretions. This is an important specific immune defence to prevent the establishment of infection

Other strategies under consideration include the use of bioadhesives such as chitosan, administered along with the surface protein influenza virus vaccine by the intranasal route, in order to facilitate uptake of the viral proteins into the cells of the respiratory tract and any local immune system cells that may be present, thereby enhancing the immune response. On a more futuristic note, the topical application of an adjuvanted influenza virus vaccine to the skin, which is rich in immunocompetent cells, particularly dendritic cells, has been the subject of recent consideration and experimentation.

Novel vaccines

All commercially available influenza virus vaccines, whether whole inactivated virus preparations or consisting of only the surface HA and NA antigens of the viruses as used in the UK, are aimed at promoting circulating or local antibodies against these surface antigens for protection against infection by the Type A and B influenza viruses. While such a strategy will be reasonably successful in stimulating effective immunity against infection by the less variable Type B influenza viruses (within the constraints on the efficacy of the host defence mechanisms), these vaccines, relying as they do on their surface proteins for promoting protection, will be far less effective against the highly variable Type A influenza viruses. This, of course, is the reason why it is necessary to update the Type A influenza virus surface antigens present in these commercially available vaccines on an almost annual basis.

However, reliance on the two major Type A influenza surface antigens as the primary protective vaccine strategy against infection by these viruses is not the sole approach to the control of this infection. Over the past decade or so, there has been considerably accelerating research, fuelled by burgeoning genetic engineering procedures and nucleic acid technology, into alternative vaccine strategies. Some such novel strategies focus on the internal, and even the non-structural, proteins of the virus, which, unlike the surface HA and NA proteins are essentially invariable between the many strains of Type A influenza virus. In recent years, the third Type A influenza virus membrane protein, the very small, highly conserved M_2 membrane protein (see Figure 1.1), has become the subject of intensive research, and a so-called 'universal' Type A influenza virus vaccine, based on the M_2 protein, that (in theory at least), does not require regular updating and therefore annual administration, is currently undergoing preclinical testing. This experimental M_2 vaccine, like the highly successful *Haemophilus influenzae* type b (Hib) vaccine, is a peptide conjugate preparation in which the outer domain of the M_2 peptide is linked to a much larger protein that imparts antigenic properties to the otherwise non-antigenic M_2 peptide domain. The rationale of this approach is that the M_2 protein plays a crucial role in viral replication, causing dissociation of the viral ribonucleoprotein (RNP), permitting this to migrate to the nucleus and continue the replication process. A number of studies using this experimental vaccine in mice, ferrets and monkeys have already indicated the potential of this approach.

Use of vaccines in general practice

Although repeated annual vaccination against influenza has been a controversial issue in the past, it now appears this strategy has an overall beneficial effect rather than a neutral one. Furthermore, there is no available evidence of any detrimental effect of annual vaccination on either the immune response levels achieved or the degree of protection afforded by the vaccine. In addition, healthcare workers have reported that current vaccines can reduce the hospitalization and mortality rates of elderly individuals with complications of influenza by approximately 50%.

A comprehensive meta-analysis, completed in 1995 by Gross *et al*, looked at 20 cohort observational studies in over 5000 elderly persons ranging in age from 65 to 101 years over a time period from 1968 to 1989. The study included three case-control studies, two cost-effectiveness studies and one randomized, double-blind, placebo-controlled study. Gross *et al* reported that vaccination of the elderly with conventional, inactivated influenza vaccine reduced the risks of pneumonia, hospitalization and death from infection by the influenza virus. Specifically, the pooled estimates of influenza vaccine efficacy indicated that vaccination of the elderly reduced:

- death rate by 68%
- hospitalization by 50%
- pneumonia by 53%
- repiratory illness by 56%.

Gross *et al* concluded that influenza immunization is an indispensable part of the care of people aged 65 years or above and that all physicians and public health organizations should be made aware of this.

A 1995 report in the *Lancet* by Karl Nicholson's group (Ahmed *et al* 1995) shows that repeated annual vaccination of the elderly is beneficial, as it reduces mortality in this group by 75%. This compares with a reduction of only 9% among persons in this cohort who receive the influenza vaccine for the first time. More recent reports by Keitel *et al* in 1997 and Beyer *et al* in 1999 indicate that the immune responses achieved following repeated annual immunization against influenza is at least as effective as that seen following a single vaccination. However, most workers agree that, in the population as a whole, the protection rates achieved in any given year by the surface protein influenza virus vaccines range from 60% to 80%

> Repeated annual vaccination of the elderly can reduce mortality by up to 75%

A more recent meta-analysis of clinical trials by Beyer *et al*, completed in 2001, and published in 2002, compared certain experimental, live attenuated influenza virus vaccines against conventional inactivated influenza virus vaccines in over 2000 people of all ages. From the five studies in this meta-analysis, it was found that efficacy, as determined by laboratory-confirmed diagnosis of influenza virus infection following either experimental challenge with wild-type influenza virus or natural challenge during an epidemic of influenza, ranged from 68% to 100%, with a mean of 78.2%. In four of these five studies, there was either an identical or a very close match between the influenza antigens present in the vaccine and those carried by the virus used for the experimental challenge or by the virus naturally in circulation in the community (Figure 7.2).

The recommendation for annual administration of influenza virus vaccine is a burden for the community-residing vaccine recipient and the individual in a long-term residential care home, in terms of having an injection and making a visit to the GP. In addition, the annual autumn vaccination programme against influenza in the UK creates an extremely heavy workload for the community and district nursing staff. At this time of year, their workload may already be increased for other reasons. Nurses have to visit patients unable to get to health centres and vaccinate residents in long-term accommodation homes.

Immunization rates

Across the UK, GP policies and rates for immunization against influenza vary widely. In a 1998 survey of influenza virus vaccination in primary care in central southern England, when national guidelines only advised immunization for individuals with specified high-risk medical conditions or for those residing in long-stay care facilities, only 11.5% overall and 64% of those over 75 years of age had been immunized against influenza. Currently available commercial influenza virus vaccines have not been popular with physicians in the UK. In a survey of 477 geriatricians in 1990, only 3% reported offering influenza vaccine to all their continuing care patients; 81% never used the vaccine. Of the 385 consultants who did not offer the vaccine, it was regarded as unnecessary by 56%, ineffective by 33% and too expensive for blanket use by 12%.

At present, GPs are reimbursed for vaccinating individuals in the 'at-risk' groups and can

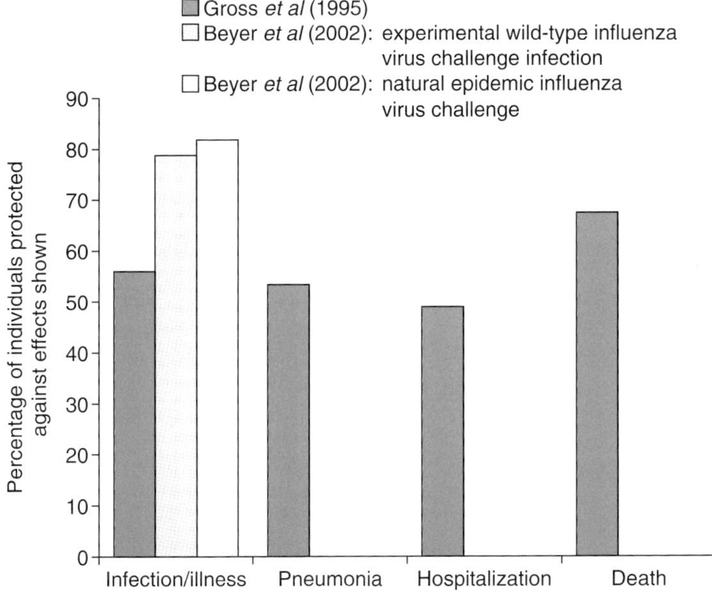

Figure 7.2
The percentages of individuals protected against infection or illness, pneumonia, hospitalization or death following immunization with conventional inactivated influenza vaccines as reported in two meta-analyses by Gross *et al* (1995) and Beyer *et al* (2002).

purchase influenza vaccine at a good discount. Nevertheless, a small-scale survey carried out over the winter of 1999/2000, covering 76 general practices within the Merton, Sutton and Wandsworth Health Authority, indicated an overall influenza vaccination rate of only 50% in those aged over 75 years. The range within individual practices was 7–97%. The study indicated that those practices achieving high coverage rates undertook personalized patient invitation and had well-organized clinics. From the year 2000, GPs have received payments for vaccinating individuals aged 65 years or older. This may well have improved the coverage of influenza vaccination in this group of the population. Indeed, preliminary data from the Merton, Sutton and Wandsworth Health Authority suggest that all the practices surveyed increased their influenza vaccine coverage the following year. The overall immunization rate for the winter of 2000/01 was 62%, thereby meeting the required government coverage target for that year of 60%.

General perception

The regular outbreaks and epidemics of influenza, coupled with the widespread non-scientific and adverse press coverage of these events, are major factors that have given rise to the belief in both the general public and those charged with delivery of the vaccine that immunization against influenza has very little effect on the course of the disease. Of course, at the population level, and as an epidemic takes hold and progresses, it is very easy to deride the effects of vaccination. However, despite the ongoing changes in the influenza viruses on an almost yearly basis, the predictions of which strains to include in the vaccine for any given year are becoming increasingly more accurate. In the current interpandemic state, where there has been no major antigenic change in the Type A influenza viruses for many years, (although this may change in the near future), vaccination is:

- saving lives
- reducing hospital admissions
- modifying the severity and duration of illness
- providing full protection against infection at the level of the individual.

Such information is derived from the annual data on the incidence of influenza in vaccinated and unvaccinated individuals gathered from well-conducted clinical trials and epidemiological studies.

However, this trend has not yet totally dispelled the concept that vaccination against influenza is a waste of time and money. This is partly because of the current inability to distinguish between true influenza virus infection and the 'influenza-like illnesses'. The latter are primarily caused by respiratory syncytial virus (RSV), parainfluenza viruses and *Mycoplasma pneumoniae*.

One comment often received by GPs from people who are to be given the influenza injection is 'I had the 'flu jab two years ago and I still had 'flu twice that winter'. This can be countered with statements to the effect that, besides influenza, there are a number of viruses and bacteria circulating in the community during winter that can cause very bad colds resembling 'flu (the 'influenza-like illnesses'), but these are not normally quite as severe as influenza nor are they normally life-threatening. Influenza can be very serious, and the influenza vaccine only protects against influenza not against these other winter respiratory tract illnesses.

Another question the physician may often be confronted with is 'Will the 'flu jab make me ill?' The response is that it will not, as it is both a safe and a non-infectious preparation. In very few recipients of the vaccine, there may be a soreness at the site of injection that lasts a few hours; in even fewer recipients, there may be a slight fever and headache, but these should last no more than 24 hours. It is now also clear that the GP can safely say that the vaccine is now known to have a beneficial effect in preventing or ameliorating illness in people in the 'at-risk' groups.

Further reading

Ahmed AH, Nicholson KG. The efficacy of influenza vaccine. *Rev Med Microbiol* 1996; **7**: 23–30.

Ahmed AE, Nicholson KG, Nguyen-Van Tam JS. Reduction in mortality associated with influenza vaccine during the 1989–90 epidemic. *Lancet* 1995; **346**: 591–5.

Beyer WE, De Bruijn IA, Palache AM *et al.* Protection against influenza after annually repeated vaccination: a meta-analysis of serologic and field studies. *Arch Intern Med* 1999 25; **159**: 182–8.

Beyer WE, Palache AM, de Jong JC, Osterhaus AD. Cold-adapted live influenza vaccine versus inactivated vaccine: systemic vaccine reactions, local and systemic antibody responses and vaccine efficacy. A meta-analysis. *Vaccine* 2002; **20**: 1340–53.

Brydak LB, Machala M. Humoral immune response to influenza vaccination in patients from high-risk groups. *Drugs* 2000; **60**: 35–53.

Carman WF, Elder AG, Wallace LA, McAulay K *et al.* Effects of influenza vaccination of health-care workers on mortality of elderly people in long-term care: a randomized controlled trial. *Lancet* 2000; **355**: 93–7.

De Bruijn IA, Remarque EJ, Jol-van der Zijde CM *et al.* Quality and quantity of humoral immune response in healthy elderly and young subjects after annually repeated influenza vaccination. *J Infect Dis* 1999; **179**: 31–6.

Eyles JE, Williamson ED, Alpar HO. Intranasal administration of influenza vaccines. *Biodrugs* 2000; **13**: 35–59.

De Filette M, Min Jou W, Birkett A *et al.* Universal influenza A vaccine: optimization of M_2-based constructs. *Virology* 2005; **337**: 149–61.

Govaert TM, Thijs CT, Sprenger MW *et al.* The efficacy of influenza vaccination in elderly individuals. A randomized double-blind placebo controlled trial. *JAMA* 1994; **272**: 1661–5.

Gross PA, Hermogenes AW, Sacks HS *et al.* The efficacy of influenza vaccine in elderly persons. A meta-analysis and review of the literature. *Ann Intern Med* 1995; **123**: 518–27.

Hall GH. Antiflu or antideath vaccination. *Lancet* 2001; **357**: 2141.

Halperin SA, Smith B, Mabrouk T *et al.* Safety and immunogenicity of a trivalent, inactivated, mammalian cell culture-driven influenza vaccine in healthy adults, seniors and children. *Vaccine* 2002; **20**: 1240–7.

Keitel WA, Cate TR, Couch RB *et al.* Efficacy of repeated annual immunization with inactivated influenza virus vaccines over a five year period. *Vaccine*. 1997; **15**: 1114–22.

Laver WG, Valentine RC. Morphology of the isolated haemagglutinin and neuraminidase subunits of influenza virus. *Virology* 1969; **38**: 105–19.

Lavanchy D. The importance of global surveillance of influenza. *Vaccine* 1999; **17**: S24–5.

Liddle BJ, Jennings R. Influenza vaccination in old age. *Age Ageing* 2001; **30**: 385–9.

Nichol KL. Clinical effectiveness and cost effectiveness of influenza vaccination among healthy working adults. *Vaccine* 1999: **17**: S67–73.

Nichol KL, Margolis KL, Wuorenma J, von Sternberg T. The efficacy and cost effectiveness of vaccination against influenza among elderly persons living in the community. *N Engl J Med* 1994; **331**: 778–84.

Ozaki T,Yauchi M, Xin K-Q et al. Cross-reactive protection against influenza A virus by a topically applied DNA vaccine encoding M gene with adjuvant. *Viral Immunol* 2005; **18**: 373–80.

Pau MG, Ophorst C, Koldijk MH et al. The human cell line PER.C6 provides a new manufacturing system for the production of influenza vaccines. *Vaccine* 2001; **19**: 2716–21.

Read RC, Naylor SC, Potter CW et al. Effective nasal vaccine delivery using chitosan. *Vaccine* 2005; **23**: 4367–74.

Snacken R. Control of influenza. Public health policies. *Vaccine* 1999; **17**(Suppl 3): S61–3.

8. Antiviral drugs for treatment and prevention

Amantadine and rimantadine
Neuraminidase inhibitors
Prophylaxis

Some drugs are now available for treatment and prevention of infection by the influenza virus, and these are summarized in Table 8.1.

Amantadine and rimantadine

The older agents amantadine and rimantadine are related substances that act by blocking the ion channel function of the influenza virus M_2 protein. This protein, although a minor surface constituent of the virus particle, is essential for viral replication. When functioning as an ion channel, the M_2 protein facilitates the entry of H+ ions into the virus particle, allowing further stages of the virus replication to proceed, as described in Chapter 7 (under 'Novel vaccines').

Amantadine and rimantadine are active against Type A influenza, but not against Type B. Both agents are effective for the treatment of Type A influenza virus infection if treatment is begun within 48 hours of the onset of illness. They can shorten the illness by approximately 1 day. Both drugs are given orally and can cause nausea and vomiting in a small percentage of individuals. Unfortunately, amantadine is associated with certain unpleasant central nervous system side-effects, such as:

- anxiety
- depression
- insomnia
- hallucinations.

These side-effects are dose-related and will resolve with discontinuation of the drug. Antiviral resistance can develop rapidly during the use of either drug, and the resistant virus can then be transmitted from the index case to others.

Although these drugs are effective, their use in clinical influenza treatment has been limited as a result of their side-effect profile. Therefore, they have not been deployed for the treatment of community-acquired influenza, but they have been used extensively in chemoprophylaxis.

Amantadine and rimantadine are:

- both effective for treatment of Type A influenza virus infection if treatment is begun within 48 hours of the onset of illness
- not active against Type B infections
- effective prophylactic agents against influenza
- relatively cheap
- liable to give rise to resistant virus strains

Neuraminidase inhibitors

Recently, neuraminidase (NA) inhibitors have been developed that have a potent anti-influenza activity *in vitro* and also have clinical efficacy. They are active against both Types A and B influenza viruses. The NA surface protein of the virus is essential for the de-aggregation and release of newly synthesized virions from infected cells. Inhibition of this enzyme interrupts propagation of the influenza virus within the human respiratory tract. Specifically, NA inhibitors are neuraminic (sialic) acid analogues, mimicking the structure of *N*-acetylneuraminic acid (Neu5Ac, NANA). This complex sugar molecule is a component of the membrane of cells susceptible to influenza virus infection. It is probably also incorporated into the lipid envelopes of the virus particles as they are released from the host cells. NANA is an important membrane structure in the final stages of influenza virus replication, and virus interaction with the NA inhibitors both diverts and blocks their reactivity with NANA.

Table 8.1
Antiviral agents for influenza

Generic name	*Trade name*	*Manufacturer*	*Influenza spectrum (Type)*	*Route of administration*	*Daily adult dosage (mg)*		*Most common side-effects*
					Prevention	*Treatment*	
Amantadine	Symmetrel	Endo Pharmaceuticals (USA)	A	Oral	200	200	Gastrointestinal and CNS
	Lysovir	Alliance (UK)					
Rimantadine†	Flumadine	Forest Laboratories (USA)	A	Oral	200	200	Gastrointestinal
Zanamivir	Relenza	GlaxoSmithKline	A and B	Oral inhalation	10	20	None
Oseltamivir	Tamiflu	Roche	A and B	Oral	75	150	Gastrointestinal

†Not available in the UK
CNS, central nervous system

Only two drugs have so far been developed to the level of entry into the formulary:

- Zanamivir is a modification of Neu5Ac2en, a dehydrated neuraminic acid derivative.
- Oseltamivir is a similar molecule, except that it has a cyclohexene ring and a polyglycerol moiety is replaced with a lipophilic side-chain.

Zanamivir can only be administered by inhalation, whereas oseltamivir can be taken by mouth. Both drugs are active against both the Type A and B influenza viruses. The structures and characteristics of oseltamivir and zanamivir are shown in Figure 8.1.

> Zanamivir and oseltamivir are effective against Types A and B influenza viruses

Efficacy

Both zanamivir and oseltamivir have been shown to be effective in the treatment of experimental Type A influenza virus infection in human studies. Both have also been shown to have significant antiviral effects in experimental Type B influenza infection. These trials are generally conducted in individuals who are susceptible to influenza virus infection – as evidenced by low titres of antibodies to influenza virus HA in the circulation.

Following intranasal inoculation with influenza virus, untreated controls suffer fever and nasopharyngeal and otological manifestations of influenza virus infection. Furthermore, proinflammatory cytokines can be measured in nasal fluids taken from these individuals. Both zanamivir and oseltamivir reduce the incidence of these symptoms when used as prophylaxis in such trials. Both drugs prevent the shedding of virus and also infection-related respiratory illness. When used in experimental treatment (ie when the drug is administered after the onset of symptoms), both drugs reduce symptom scores and duration of illness.

Treatment of community-acquired influenza

Some clinical trials have been published regarding the use of zanamivir and oseltamivir in the treatment of patients with influenza in the community (Table 8.2).

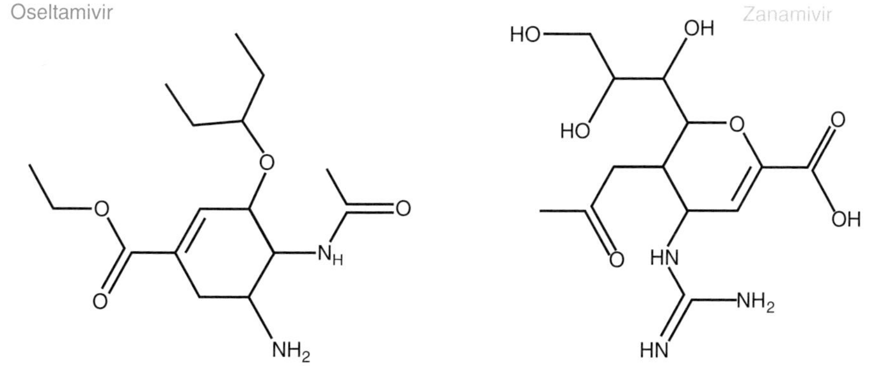

Oseltamivir

Oral absorption: 75%
Plasma $t_{1/2}$: 7–9 hours
Dosage: adults 75–150 mg/day
Toxicity: nausea in 10% alleviated by food
Acquired resistance: rare
Capsules and suspension

Zanamivir

Poor oral bioavailability
After inhalation, excellent mucosal levels
Dosage: 10 mg inhaled powder twice daily
Toxicity: cough/bronchoconstriction occur
Acquired resistance: rare <1%
Dry powder for inhalation

Figure 8.1
Structure and characteristics of oseltamivir and zanamivir.

Table 8.2
Neuraminidase inhibitors in the treatment of community-acquired influenza

Treatment	*Patients (% with proven influenza)*	*Age range (mean)*	*Duration of illness*	*Median reduction in days to alleviation of symptoms in patients with influenza*	*Comments*	*Investigators*
Inhaled zanamivir 10 mg bid for 5 days	417 (63%)	≥13 years (32 years)	≤48 hours	1 (5 vs 4) 3 (7 vs 4 in febrile)	3 days reduction in patients treated <30 hours	Hayden *et al* (1997)
Inhaled zanamivir 10 mg bid for 5 days	455 (71%)	≥12 years (37 years)	<30 hours	1.5 (6.5 vs 5.0)	Reduced complications and antibiotics (15% vs 38%) in patients with underlying conditions. No effect in patients with symptoms >30 hours	MIST Study Group (1998)
			>30 hours	2.0 (6.5 vs 4.5 in febrile)		
Oseltamivir 75 mg or 150 mg bid for 5 days	629 (60%)	18–65 years	≤36 hours	1.4 (4.3 vs 2.9 vs 2.9)	Reduced complications	Treanor *et al* (2000)
Oseltamivir 75 mg or 150 mg bid for 5 days	719 (66%)	18–65 years	≤36 hours	1.2–1.5 days (4.9 vs 3.6 vs 3.4)	No difference between doses	Nicholson *et al* (2000)
Oseltamivir 75 mg bid for 5 days	1426 (67%)	12–70 years	<6 hours <12 hours <24 hours <36 hours	3.5 days 3.1 days 2.3 days 1.2 days	Earlier administration reduced symptoms still further	Aoki *et al* (2003)

The evidence yielded by these studies has recently been reviewed by the Cochrane Collaboration. NA inhibitors have been shown to shorten the duration of symptoms by 1 day. Across all studies, the time gained in returning to normal activities is half a day for laboratory-confirmed cases of influenza. The beneficial effect appears to be confined to patients in whom there is fever, and who are treated within 30 hours of the onset of symptoms. NA inhibitors reduce the frequency of complications of influenza. In children who have influenza-like illness, oseltamivir has been shown to reduce the likelihood of acute otitis media. The use of oseltamivir reduces the need for hospitalization of adults with influenza and is associated with less antibiotic use. More recently, in an open-label, muticentre international study among over 1400 patients undertaken during the winter season of 1999–2000, and reported in 2003, Aoki and colleagues of the IMPACT group found that the commencement of treatment with oseltamivir (75 mg twice daily for 5 days) within the first 12 hours after the onset of fever significantly reduced the duration of illness by just over 3 days compared with the duration of illness recorded when treatment was commenced later, at 48 hours after the onset of fever (Table 8.2).

So far, the NA inhibitors have not been extensively investigated in patients who are at the highest risk of serious complications of influenza. Such patients include the elderly and those with serious cardiopulmonary illness, such as chronic obstructive pulmonary disease. Although oseltamivir can be given orally, zanamivir must be given via an inhaler device – it is possible that both older and very young patients may not be able to deliver the drug effectively by this method.

Both drugs appear relatively safe. Zanamivir has very few side-effects, but there is significant incidence of nausea with oseltamivir. However, this is generally associated with the first dose only, is transient in nature and is reduced when the drug is taken with food. When used for the treatment of children, inhaled zanamivir significantly reduced the time to alleviation of illness (by approximately 1 day). It has also reduced the time required for return to normal activities. Nebulized zanamivir is available for the treatment of younger children and infants. A liquid formulation of oseltamivir is effective in children aged between 1 and 10 years, and it reduces the frequency of complications leading to antibiotic prescriptions.

Neuraminidase inhibitors have not yet been extensively investigated in patients who are at the highest risk of serious complications of influenza

Prophylaxis

Antiviral agents are valuable alternatives to vaccines for augmenting protection among vulnerable individuals, particularly patients who are immunodeficient. They are also very useful in the prevention of influenza within households and in institutional settings such as long-term care facilities for the elderly. Protection against infection is particularly important for:

- unvaccinated high-risk persons (the elderly or those with cardiopulmonary disease)
- high-risk persons when the vaccine–epidemic virus match is poor
- vaccinated persons during the window period after vaccination (10–14 days)
- unvaccinated healthcare workers
- staff in long-term care facilities during an influenza epidemic.

Studies conducted over many years have shown that amantadine and rimantadine are very effective as prophylactic agents for the control of Type A influenza virus infections in nursing care facilities. Development of resistance in this circumstance has not been a particular problem. Amantadine and rimantadine are relatively cheap drugs, which makes them preferred agents in this indication.

Both oseltamivir and zanamivir have been shown to prevent influenza, and their use in

Table 8.3
Neuraminidase inhibitors in chemoprophylaxis

Drug	*No. of subjects*	*Exposure*	*Intervention*	*Outcome measurement*	*Result*	*Comments*	*Investigators*
Zanamivir (Zm)	575	Close community contacts	Intranasal Zm (10 mg), inhaled Zm, or both in intranasal and inhaled Zm or placebo for 5 days	Rate of influenza contacts	Inhaled Zm reduced influenza rate	Intranasal Zm was ineffective	Kaiser *et al* (2000)
Zanamivir (Zm)	837	Family or household contacts	Inhaled Zm (10 mg) to household contacts of influenza cases or placebo for 5 days	Proportion of households with a secondary case	Zm reduced households with secondary cases: 19% placebo versus 4% Zm	No Zm resistance emerged	Hayden *et al* (2000)
Oseltamivir (Os)	955	Family or household contacts	Oseltamivir orally (75 mg) or placebo for 7 days	Rate of secondary clinical influenza in individuals and households	Os significantly reduced secondary cases and rates of secondary household infections. Viral shedding also reduced in contacts	Os side-effects similar to placebo	Welliver *et al* (2001)
Oseltamivir (Os)	236	Nursing home residents during natural Type B influenza index residential epidemic	Oseltamivir (75 mg) orally for 7 days	Secondary case rate compared with historical control without oseltamivir	Secondary case rate reduced from 19% to 10%	No placebo	Parker *et al* (2001)

chemoprophylaxis has been reviewed by the Cochrane Collaboration.

Influenza virus NA inhibitors, when compared with placebo, are 74% effective in preventing naturally occurring cases of clinically defined influenza (95% confidence interval (CI) 50–87%), and 60% effective in preventing cases of laboratory-confirmed influenza virus infection (95% CI 76–33%). Several placebo-controlled studies of zanamivir and oseltamivir have now been conducted (Table 8.3).

NA inhibitors have been administered to close contacts of index cases within 48 hours of initial clinical infection. Outcome measurements have included the infection rate in individual contacts, or the proportion of households in which new cases have been proven using laboratory methods. Zanamivir and oseltamivir appear to be equally effective and are of similar cost (considerably higher than that of amantadine). However, ease of administration favours the use of oseltamivir in the context of long-term care facilities. Administration of zanamivir requires good hand–eye coordination, lung function and comprehension. In the future, if NA inhibitors become licensed for this indication, they would probably be administered for 7–14 days in prophylactic situations.

With the increased understanding of the events involved in the growth and replication of influenza viruses at the molecular and cellular level, and the increased awareness of the interactions of the virus with a variety of host cell defence mechanisms, there is hope that the rate of discovery of new anti-influenza drugs will both continue and amplify. The NICE guidelines for the prophylaxis of influenza are shown in Table 8.4.

Table 8.4
NICE guidance to NHS: amantadine and oseltamivir for prophylaxis of influenza

When Type A or B influenza circulates in community:

- Oseltamivir is recommended for post-exposure prophylaxis for at-risk individuals aged >13 years if they can begin drug <48 hours post exposure, if they live in residential care, whether or not they have been vaccinated
- Oseltamivir is recommended for the same group in the community, if they are unvaccinated
- Oseltamivir is not recommmended for use in healthy persons aged <65, or as seasonal prophylaxis
- Amantadine is not recommended

Further reading

Aoki FY, MacLeod MD, Paggiaro P *et al.* Early administration of oral oseltamivir increases the benefits of influenza treatment. *J Antimicrob Chemother* 2003; **51**: 123–9.

Gubareva LV, Kaiser L, Hayden FG. Influenza virus neuraminidase inhibitors. *Lancet* 2000; **355**: 827–35.

Hayden FG. Amantadine and rimantadine – clinical aspects. In: Richman DD (ed). *Antiviral Drug Resistance.* Chichester: Wiley, 1996: 59–71.

Hayden FG, Osterhaus AD, Treanor JJ *et al.* Efficacy and safety of the neuraminidase inhibitor zanamivir in the treatment of influenzavirus infections. GG167 Influenza Study Group. *N Engl J Med* 1997; **337**: 874–80.

Hayden FG, Gubareva LV, Monto AS, *et al.* Inhaled zanamivir for the prevention of influenza in families. Zanamivir Family Study Group. *N Engl J Med* 2000; **343**: 1282–9.

Jefferson T, Demicheli V, Deeks J, Rivetti D. Neuraminidase inhibitors for preventing and treating influenza in healthy adults (Cochrane Review). In: *The Cochrane Library*, Issue 1. Oxford: Update Software, 2002.

Kaiser L, Henry D, Flack NP *et al.* Short-term treatment with zanamivir to prevent influenza: results of a placebo-controlled study. *Clin Infect Dis* 2000; **30**: 587–9.

MIST (Management of Influenza in the Southern Hemisphere Trialists) Study Group. Randomised trial of efficacy and safety of inhaled zanamivir in treatment of influenza A and B virus infections. *Lancet* 1998; **352**: 1877–81.

Nicholson KG, Aoki FY, Osterhaus AD *et al.* Efficacy and safety of oseltamivir in treatment of acute influenza: a randomized controlled trial. Neuraminidase Inhibitor Flu Treatment Investigator Group. *Lancet* 2000; **355**: 1845–50.

Parker R, Loewen N, Skowronski D. Experience with oseltamivir in the control of a nursing home influenza B outbreak. *Can Commun Dis Rep* 2001; **27**: 37–40.

Treanor JJ, Hayden FG, Vrooman PS *et al.* Efficacy and safety of the oral neuraminidase inhibitor oseltamivir in treating acute influenza: a randomized controlled trial. US Oral Neuraminidase Study Group. *JAMA* 2000; **283**: 1016–24.

Welliver R, Monto AS, Carewicz O *et al.* Effectiveness of oseltamivir in preventing influenza in household contact: a randomized controlled trial. *JAMA* 2001; **285**: 748–54.

9. Management

Immunization
Diagnosis
Standard treatment
Complications
The workplace

Immunization

In the early autumn of every year, all GPs in the UK initiate immunization programmes for influenza. Currently, UK government policy is to recommend influenza immunization for:

- all people aged 65 years and over
- people of all ages with chronic respiratory or heart disease, renal disease or diabetes mellitus
- all those who are immunocompromised
- all persons living in long-stay residential accommodation.

The question of whether to immunize a given individual rests entirely with the GP. However, targets are currently set by the government and monitored by the primary care organizations. In 2001, an overall nationwide target uptake of influenza immunization for individuals aged 65 years and above was set at 70%, with the aim of achieving a minimum uptake of 65%. The vaccine is given by intramuscular injection, and some vaccine recipients experience some local pain from this injection. There may also be some temporary soreness at the injection site that lasts 24–48 hours. Other side-effects are very rare, but include fever and muscle aches, which can last up to 2 days.

It is impossible for influenza vaccine to cause influenza, as it does not contain live virus – it contains only proteins derived from the virus. In some parts of the world, the vaccine used contains intact but killed virus, which will also not cause influenza. The vaccine is contraindicated for people with severe allergy to hen's eggs, as the vaccine is manufactured in eggs and minute traces of egg protein may remain despite purification. Further information regarding vaccination on an annual basis is available on the Department of Health website (see the list of useful websites at the end of this book).

> It is impossible for influenza vaccine to cause influenza

The clinically compromised groups at special risk from influenza virus infection, who are therefore targeted for influenza vaccination, are outlined in Chapter 7. However, such is their importance that they are described more fully in Table 9.1.

Diagnosis

The clinical diagnosis of influenza virus infection is extremely difficult outside the influenza season, as many respiratory tract infections can mimic influenza. Even in the winter, if no clear-cut epidemic is evident, the infection may be difficult to diagnose on clinical grounds alone. In general, an 'influenza-like illness' is recognized as an abrupt onset of fever and chills accompanied by:

- headache
- sore throat
- myalgias
- malaise
- anorexia
- dry cough.

The fever, which peaks within 24–48 hours of onset, can last from 1 to 5 days. Physical signs include:

- a hot and moist face
- flushing
- subconjunctival suffusion

Table 9.1
Risk groups for influenza immunization

General condition	Examples
Chronic respiratory disease, including asthma	• Chronic obstructive pulmonary disease (COPD) • Chronic bronchitis and emphysema • Cystic fibrosis • Interstitial lung fibrosis • Pneumoconiosis • Asthma requiring continuous or repeated use of inhaled or systemic steroids • Asthma with previous exacerbations requiring hospital admission
Chronic heart disease	• Chronic ischaemic heart disease • Congenital heart disease and hypertensive heart disease requiring regular medication and follow-up (but excluding uncomplicated controlled hypertension) • Chronic heart failure
Chronic renal disease	• Nephrotic syndrome • Chronic renal failure • Renal transplantation patients
Diabetes	• Diabetes mellitus requiring insulin or oral hypoglycaemic drugs
Immunosuppression	• Due to disease or treatment, including systemic steroids equivalent to 20 mg prednisolone daily for >2 weeks (Some immunocompromised patients may have a suboptimal immunological response to the vaccine)

Derived from Department of Health. Current vaccine and immunization issues 2001, P/L/CMO/2001/1

- reddened nasal and mucosal surfaces
- clear nasal discharge.

In addition, adults occasionally have arthralgia, abdominal pain, chest pain and cervical lymphadenopathy. Children may also present with the features of a non-specific febrile illness, or with a respiratory illness such as croup, bronchiolitis or bronchitis. These are very similar to the diseases caused by parainfluenza viruses and respiratory syncytial virus (RSV).

During the influenza season (December–March), baseline rates of influenza can rise from below 50 cases to between 50 and 400 cases per 100 000 individuals each week. An influenza epidemic is defined as more than 400 cases per 100 000 of the population per week. Figure 1.4 shows the pattern of influenza activity in the UK over the years 1988 to 2000.

In practice, it is impossible for GPs to distinguish influenza virus infection from other respiratory tract infections, with certainty, on clinical grounds alone. Influenza viruses account for only about one-half of the influenza-like illness seen by GPs during the influenza season; the other pathogens involved being RSV, parainfluenza viruses, some picornaviruses and *Mycoplasma pneumoniae*. Although 'near-patient testing' technologies are being developed, these currently lack the required sensitivity and specificity necessary for widespread deployment. Near-patient testing involves bedside tests that do not require samples to be sent to the laboratory. Therefore GPs are still required to make a diagnosis on purely clinical grounds, and, in the absence of laboratory confirmation, this diagnosis is as an influenza-like illness.

Laboratory diagnosis is not normally carried out on a routine basis. At the start of the influenza season in the UK, as cases of influenza-like illness begin to appear in a community, the Health Protection Agency is involved in confirming the infection as influenza in a small proportion of these initial 'index' cases. This is not only to register the presence and activity of the virus in the area, but also to determine if the circulating virus is a Type A or Type B virus. If it is a Type A virus, it is important to know whether it is an H3N2 or H1N1 subtype.

Laboratory diagnosis

As indicated above, not until near-patient testing technology becomes routine practice will it become possible to distinguish clinical influenza from influenza-like illnesses with certainty. Nevertheless, during the influenza season, and in the presence of both a confirmed epidemic in the country and laboratory-confirmed cases of influenza in the community, an individual experiencing an abrupt onset of respiratory tract symptoms accompanied by malaise, headache, myalgia in the back and limbs, and a temperature of 38–40°C could be presumptively diagnosed as suffering from an influenza virus infection.

Although laboratory diagnosis is not normally sought for most cases of influenza, if hospitalization of a patient with suspected influenza infection becomes necessary, the infection must be diagnosed by the laboratory. In practice, the presence of the virus is best confirmed using nasopharyngeal aspirates. These may be collected using suction and trap methods in the hospital laboratory. In the doctor's surgery, throat swabs or preferably nasal washings may be taken if nasopharyngeal aspirates cannot be obtained. Throat swabs are, in general, not as effective as nasal washings for laboratory diagnosis of influenza. All samples for laboratory diagnosis must be placed into appropriate virus-preserving fluid medium, stored (for the minimum time possible) at 4°C and transported to the laboratory on ice as quickly as possible. Routine methods of laboratory testing for influenza virus include:

- examination for specific viral antigens by fluorescent microscopy
- cultivation of the virus in embryonated hen's eggs
- occasional cultivation of the virus in tissue culture.

> Nasal washes are more effective than throat swabs in the diagnosis of influenza in the laboratory

Diagnostic technologies for influenza virus that are still at the experimental stage and not yet available for routine use include the polymerase chain reaction (PCR) to specifically detect the viral nucleic acid.

Blood samples are usually taken at the onset of illness. However, the laboratory diagnosis of influenza virus infection by serological methods can only be made on collection of a second blood sample from the patient at convalescence. Both samples are tested simultaneously to demonstrate a significant rise in the level of specific antibodies to the influenza virus in the convalescent sample. Such laboratory diagnosis is necessarily retrospective and is therefore of epidemiological rather than clinical significance.

Standard treatment

The management of influenza in individual patients entails both symptomatic treatment and the use of the novel antiviral agents that are becoming increasingly available. All patients with influenza should be encouraged to:

- drink adequate fluids
- take paracetamol to reduce symptoms
- stay off work
- rest at home in bed
- take appropriate antivirals as indicated by the Health Protection Agency.

The nature and mechanisms of action of the antiviral agents operating against influenza are dealt with in Chapter 8. In practice, the neuraminidase inhibitors, which include zanamivir and oseltamivir, are the only drugs that can modify the natural history of influenza virus infection without causing unacceptable side-effects. The National Institute for Clinical Excellence (NICE) has provided guidance on the use of oseltamivir in the treatment of influenza.

Zanamivir and oseltamivir act against a stage of the viral replication cycle (release of virus from the infected cell) that is specific to the influenza viruses. Therefore, they have no beneficial activity against other viruses or against *M. pneumoniae*. There are also no harmful effects of these antiviral drugs should they be given to individuals suffering from an influenza-like illness.

> Patients with influenza should be encouraged to drink adequate fluids, to take paracetamol to reduce symptoms, to stay off work and to rest at home in bed

As soon as the Health Protection Agency has signalled that influenza is circulating in the community, it is recommended that oseltamivir be prescribed for 'at-risk' adults who present within 36 hours of the onset of an influenza-like illness, and who are able to commence treatment within 48 hours of the onset of these symptoms. The 'at-risk' adults are individuals falling into one or more of the categories listed in Table 7.1.

The NICE guidelines 2003 are summarized in Table 9.2.

> The neuraminidase inhibitors are the only drugs that can modify the natural history of influenza virus infection without causing unacceptable side-effects

Table 9.2
NICE guidance to NHS: zanamivir, oseltamivir and amantadine for the treatment of influenza

When Type A influenza circulates in community:

- Zanamivir and oseltamivir are not recommended for any individuals who are not at risk
- Amantadine is not recommended for treatment
- Zanamivir and oseltamivir are recommended for treatment of at-risk individuals with influenza-like illness <48 hours
- Oseltamivir is recommended for treatment of at-risk children with influenza-like illness <48 hours

Complications

Pneumonia

The most common serious complication of influenza is pneumonia – this may occur at the same time as the influenza-like illness or could arise up to 2 weeks afterwards.

- If the pneumonia appears during the influenza-like illness then it is possible that it is a primary viral pneumonia caused by the virus itself. However, this is relatively uncommon.
- If the pneumonia commences after apparent recovery from the influenza infection then it is most likely that there is a bacterial superinfection. This is usually due to either *Streptococcus pneumoniae* or, less commonly, *Staphylococcus aureus*.

All influenza virus pneumonias should be assumed to be bacterial because of the high mortality rate, particularly in the 'at-risk' groups. All patients should therefore be carefully evaluated for symptoms and signs of pneumonia. Any patient with evidence of lung consolidation should be evaluated for possible hospital admission and should be treated with antibiotics using the guidance supplied by the Health Protection Agency, the British Thoracic Society and the British Infection Society. This would include the use of co-amoxiclav or doxycycline. It is common practice to include the use of oral flucloxacillin in patients who present with pneumonia after influenza, because of the increased frequency of *S. aureus* pneumonias in this group.

GPs will advise patients with influenza to stay at home, but should remain aware of the possibility of complications arising in the patient (eg pneumonia). GPs are faced with the tension of coping with an unmanageable home-visiting load and missing a case of pneumonia. It is important that the physician can advise the patient with influenza to be aware of symptoms such as:

- shortness of breath
- pleuritic chest pain
- haemoptysis.

Any or all of these may herald the development of pneumonia. Should such symptoms arise in the patient, he or she should contact the doctor immediately.

Residential care homes

If a GP encounters a cluster of influenza-like illnesses in a nursing home or other residential facility, the initial cases should be treated as outlined above. The most important intervention is to contact the local consultant in communicable disease control. Subsequently, the public health authorities will be able to make an assessment of the risk to other residents, and institute control of infection policies, such as chemoprophylaxis, if necessary.

Bacterial infections

The complications that may follow influenza virus infection in an elderly individual, in an individual suffering from a chronic respiratory or cardiovascular condition, or very occasionally in a healthy adult are likely to be more severe than any complications that may follow an influenza-like illness. This is not only due to the almost complete destruction of the ciliated epithelial cells lining the trachea and bronchii of the respiratory tract, but is also associated with the systemic symptoms arising during influenza virus infection that, although not fully understood, seem to impose a considerable strain on the body. This interaction of the influenza virus with the host can be considerably more severe than that caused by other infectious agents that give rise to influenza-like illnesses.

However, there could be complications following infection with *M. pneumoniae*. Infection by this agent may result in a lengthy illness sometimes accompanied by clinical depression and occasional haematological and neurological sequelae. This distinguishes infection by *M. pneumoniae* from an influenza infection with complications.

There are few serious complications subsequent to RSV infection in adults, and infections by parainfluenza viruses are usually mild. In infants and young children less than 2 years of age (a group not normally victims of disease caused by the influenza virus), RSV can cause a severe, acute bronchiolitis that carries a mortality rate of 0.1% in untreated cases. Parainfluenza viruses are associated with croup (an acute laryngotracheobronchitis) in children under 5 years of age, although this infection carries no significant mortality.

The workplace

Management of influenza in the workplace centres around vaccination. When faced with an impending epidemic, some industrial companies may choose to offer their employees immunization with the current vaccine, in order to minimize sickness and absenteeism through influenza or influenza-like illness. In the special case of the essential service industries – such as the healthcare professions and the fire and police services – immunization is recommended. This is especially true where advance notice has been received of the arrival of a Type A or B influenza strain that has significant antigenic differences from preceding strains.

It must be stressed that influenza vaccination in the UK remains optional. It is at the discretion of the individual to receive the injection, and at the discretion of commercial or industrial companies to offer it.

Further reading

Boivin G, Osterhaus AD, Gaudreau A *et al.* Role of picornaviruses in flu-like illnesses of adults enrolled in an oseltamivir treatment study who had no evidence of influenza virus infection. *J Clin Microbiol* 2002; **40**: 330–4.

Furey A, Robinson E, Young Y. Improving immunisation coverage in 2000–2001: A baseline survey, review of the evidence and sharing of best practice. *Commun Dis Public Health* 2001; **4**: 183–7.

Gupta A, Morris G, Thomas P, Hasan M. Influenza vaccination coverage in old people's homes in Carmarthenshire, UK, during the winter of 1998/99. *Vaccine* 2000; **18**: 2471–5.

Gupta A, Makinde K, Morris G *et al.* Influenza immunisation coverage in older hospitalised patients during winter 1998–99 in Carmarthenshire, UK. *Age and Ageing*; **29**: 211–13.

Kumpulainen V, Makela M. Influenza among healthy employees: a cost-benefit analysis. *Scand J Infect Dis* 1997; **29**: 181–5.

Useful websites

Association of Medical Microbiologists

www.amm.co.uk/newamm/files/factsabout/fa_flu

- This website comprises three pages of basic facts about the influenza viruses and their transmission, together with a description of the clinical syndrome of influenza, its prevention and treatment.

Department of Health

www.doh.gov.uk

- This is a generally useful website with regularly updated information on topical issues and a number of links to the NHS. www.doh.gov.uk/zanamivirguidance
- This website is designed specifically to provide up-to-date information on the anti-influenza drug zanamivir, and it is primarily aimed at GPs. There is guidance on the conditions under which zanamivir can be used, sections concerned with both national and local action, and links to sites covering patient management not dealt with by the NICE recommendations for treatment of influenza.

European Scientific Working Group on influenza

www.eswi.org/intro.cfm

- This website from the European Scientific Working Group on Influenza offers updated information on influenza viruses, the disease, diagnosis, epidemiology, prevention and control. The group also issues a twice-yearly bulletin, 'Influenza', available on the website.

'Flu index page

www.hpa.org.uk/infections/topics_az/influenza/flu.htm

- This website from the Health Protection Agency is specifically concerned with accessing up-to-date information about most aspects of influenza, including 'frequently asked questions on flu', the current situation on influenza surveillance, the treatment of influenza and Health Protection Agency publications on influenza. There is also a link to related influenza websites.

Influenza vaccination

www.jr2.ox.ac.uk/bandolier/band73/b73-7.html

- This website summarizes the findings of recent clinical trials of influenza vaccines in terms of their efficacy and any documented adverse effects. It provides information on the value and effectiveness of influenza vaccines.

Morbidity statistics

www.rcgp.org.uk

- The Royal College of General Practitioners website provides weekly morbidity statistics on respiratory and influenza-like illness from general practices, as well as the results of statistical analyses on consulting patterns, age group differences and comparisons between current and previous years with respect to the incidence of influenza.

National Institute for Clinical Excellence (NICE)

www.nice.org.uk

- This comprehensive website provides a valuable starting point for accessing updated information about recent advances in the treatment of diseases, including influenza. It also includes general information about NICE and its activities, along with links to further websites on influenza.

World Health Organization (WHO)

www.who.int/topics/influenza/en/

- This website covers, through many links, basic facts about influenza, the WHO influenza programme, national pandemic preparation plans, recommendations for vaccine composition, and the use of vaccines and other preventative measures.

www.who.int/csr/disease/avian_influenza/guidelines/infectioncontrol/en/

www.who.int/csr/disease/avian_influenza/guidelines/clinicalmanage/en/

- These websites concerned are with interim infection control guidelines for health care facilities and interim guidelines on clinical management of humans infected with the H5N1 strain of Type A influenza.
- For the influenza fanatic, there is also a link to the 'Influenza Bibliography Listings', which lists all publications worldwide that touch upon the virus, the infection and its control.

Index

Page numbers in *italics* refer to information that is shown only in a table or diagram.

amantadine 55–6
  NICE guidance to NHS 61, 66
  prophylaxis 59–61
  side-effects 55
animal models of human infection 16
  destruction of ciliated epithelial cells **16**
antibodies
  correlation of HA status with type A infection **18**
  IgA, IgG, IgM 17
  imperfect match with viral antigens 9–10
  local response 17–18
  serum antibody (IgG) 18
antigenic drift 5, 9, 15, 21
antigenic shift 10–11, 21
antiviral drugs 55–61
  amantadine and rimantadine 55
  Cochrane Collaboration 59, 61
  generic and trade names 56
  neuraminidase inhibitors 55–9
  prophylaxis 59–61
  treatment of community-acquired influenza 57–8
Asia, SE
  avian influenza cross-transmission 23
  H5N1 virus 7
Asian flu epidemics 7, 11
Association of Medical Microbiologists (website) 69
asthma 40
avian (type A) influenza
  cases 2003–2006 **30**
  clinical assessment 34–5
  clinical disease 26–7
  control 27–8
  cross-species transmission 22–30
    Guangdong geese 25
    poultry to humans 22, 23
    to pigs 22, 23
  deaths 2003–2006 **30**
  epidemiology 23
  first reported 26
  H2N2 (1957) and H3N2 (1968) serotypes, and pigs 30
  H5N1 strain 22
    excretion by healthy ducks 27
  HA, NA combinations 22, 23
    spread from poultry to humans 22, 23
  pathogenicity and virulence 12, 24–6
  relationships with mammalian and human influenza viruses 21–30
  reservoir for all 15 of HA proteins/antigens 24–5
  Vietnam 34
  virulence factors 12, 24–6
    avirulent/virulent strains **26**
  waders/wildfowl, adaptation 21, 23

bacterial (secondary) complications 37–40, 67
  asthma 40
  bronchiectasis 39
  clinical features 39–40
  COPD 39
  cystic fibrosis 39
  diabetes 40
  H. influenzae, *Staph. aureus*, *Strep. pneumoniae* 37–8
  HIV infection 40
  ischaemic heart disease 40
  morbidity 38–9
  pathogenesis 38
  secondary invasion of lower respiratory tract 16
  smoking 40
bronchiectasis 39

canines, subtype H3N8 virus, cross-transmission from horses 23
cardiac myositis 32
children
  symptoms 31–2
  vectors for infection, virus shedding period 9
China
  Beijing type A virus 6
  cases and deaths 2003–2006 **30**
  cross-species transmission, H3N2 strain in pigs 24
  equine influenza, subtype H3N8 24
  Guangdong geese 25
chitosan 48
chronic heart disease 64
chronic obstructive pulmonary disease (COPD) 39
chronic renal disease 64
chronic respiratory disease including asthma 64
cilia *see* epithelial cells
clearance of virus 18–19
clinical assessment 31–5
  diagnosis 33
  influenza in pregnancy 34
  management of seasonal influenza 34
  myositis 32
  Reye's syndrome 32
  symptoms in adults 31
  symptoms in children 31–2
Cochrane Collaboration, antiviral drugs 59, 61
complications of influenza 37–41, 66–7
  bacterial disease 37–40
  immunocompromised patients 37
  pneumonia 32–3, 66–7
  in residential care homes 67
  workplaces 67
  see also bacterial (secondary) complications
control 27–8
cross-species transmission *v* 11, 22–30, **28**
  between mammals, birds and humans 29–30
  and genetic reassortment 11, 21–2
croup 67
cystic fibrosis 39
cytotoxic T cells, immune mechanisms 12–13

Department of Health (DoH), website 69
diabetes mellitus 40
  immunization 64
diagnosis of influenza 33, 63–5
  laboratory diagnosis 33, 65

eggs
  allergies 46
  see also hens' eggs for vaccine production
elderly persons
  immunization, metaanalysis 1968–1989 49–50, **51**
  mortality 37
  repeated annual vaccination 50
epidemics vs pandemics, *endmatter*
epidemiology 9–14
  antigenic drift 5, 9, 15, 21
  antigenic shift 10–11, 21
  antigenic variability 9–10
  avian influenza 23
  infection patterns 9
epithelial cells *see* respiratory tract epithelial cells
equine influenza
  in China 24
  clinical disease 27
  subtype H3N8, cross-transmission 23
  subtypes H7N7 and H3N8 24
  transmission to dogs 23
European Scientific Working Group on Influenza, website 69

felines (tigers and leopards)
  clinical disease 27
  cross-transmission of H5N1 22, 27, **28**
ferret, model of human infection 16
Flumadine *see* rimantadine
furin, intracellular endoprotease, infectivity of type A virus 25

general practice
  vaccines in general practice 49–50
  see also management
genetic reassortment
  cross-species transmission 11, 21–2
  and pandemics 11
  porcine respiratory tract as 'mixing' vessel 24
  in vaccine production 45
glycoproteins *see* haemagglutinin; neuraminidase

growth and replication 4, **5**
"budding" process **5**
Guillain-Barré syndrome 46

haemagglutinin 4–5
antigenic variability 9–10
H1, H2 and H3 serotypes 21, **22**
mutations affecting cleavage, and high virulence 24–5
in non-human species 6, **22**
novel HA protein 21
nucleotide substitution rates **7**
number (15) of HA proteins/antigens 11, 21–2
systemic antibody levels, and protection against infection 12–13
haemagglutinin gene, variation, type A vs type B **7**
Haemophilus influenzae infection 37
Health Protection Agency 64
websites, 'Flu index page 69
heart disease
bacterial complications 40
immunization 64
hens' eggs for vaccine production 45, 63
alternatives 46
egg allergies 46
Hong Kong (H3N2 subtype)
1967 pandemic 29–30
1997 epidemic 7, 11, 34–5
control measures 27
proximity to China and Guangdong geese 25
horses *see* equine influenza
host cell receptors 4
humans
as "dead-end" host 22
human/pig cross-transmission 22, 23, **28**, 30
resistance to infection 12–13

immune defence mechanisms 12–13, 18–19
cellular/humoral responses 12
clearance of virus 18–19
events with infection in respiratory tract **47**
local and systemic 48
time delay 13
immunization 43–52, 63
efficacy 43
elderly persons, metaanalysis 1968–1989 49–50, **51**
groups recommended (risk groups) 43–4, **45**, **64**
immunization rates 50–1
new strategies of vaccination 47–9
chitosan adhesive 48–9
delivery by nasal route 48
topical application 49
problems 43, 46–7
local reactions 46
safety 46, 63
vaccine immunogenicity, determination 47
vaccine production 44–6
genetic reassortment 45
novel vaccines 46, 49
strain selection by WHO 44–5
surface antigen influenza vaccine **44**
vaccines in general practice 49–50
general perception 51–2
percentages of protection acquired following immunization 51
website 69
immunocompromised patients 37–41
immunization 64
see also specfic conditions
immunological memory, primary/secondary infection 18
Indonesia 35
influenza A virus
see also influenza A virus infection
ability to establish infection 12–13
availability of host endonucleases 25
extracellular endoproteases, plasmin 25
intracellular endoproteases, furin 25
antigenic drift 5, 9, 15, 21
cross-species transmission *v* 11, 22–30
humans to/from pigs 22, 23
see also avian influenza
genetic variation 1, 5
growth and replication 4–5, 16
fusion of HA and intracellular vacuolar membrane 25
H3N2 and H1N1 current subtypes 11
H3N8, cross-transmission to dogs from horses 23
H5N1, H9N2, H7N7, H7N3 22 serotypes 22

influenza A virus – (*continued*)
H5N1 serotype
human cases of avian influenza 11, 22
limited spread between humans 22
HA molecule, cleavage 25
half-life 9
human as "dead-end" host 22
human resistance to infection 12–13
isolation from harbour seals, whales, mink **22**, 24
M_1 and M_2 proteins 5, 55
rapid evolution, causes 23
single host species infection 11
structure 3–4
subtypes **12**
surface glycoproteins 5
serotypes in mammals and birds **22**
see also haemagglutinin; neuraminidase
survival time of particles 9
titre, and antibody levels **10**
virulence factors 12
avirulent strains 25
intracellular endoprotease (furin) 25
see also avian (type A) influenza
influenza A virus infection
correlation of HA antibody status with infection **18**
frequency and duration of symptoms of Type A/Hong Kong/68 influenza virus 32
H3N2 and H1N1 subtypes, severity of illness 12
H5N1 serotype, human cases of avian influenza 22
incubation period 9
transient viraemia 15
see also influenza A virus
influenza B and C virus
genetic variation 5
vaccine production 44–6
influenza B and C virus infections
antibodies to 15
antiviral drugs 55
characteristics 7
incubation period 9
morbidity 1989–1999 **39**
influenza in non-human species 6
Influenza Surveillance Network, vaccine strain selection by WHO 44–5
influenza-like illness 31, 64
weekly consultation rates **6**
interferon 17
and virus titre **10**
ischaemic heart disease, bacterial complications 40

laboratory diagnosis 33, 65
laryngotracheobronchitis 67
latency (none?) 15
local host factors 17–18
Lysovir *see* amantadine

management 63–70
complications of influenza 66–7
neuraminidase inhibitors, treatment of community-acquired influenza 57–8
risk groups for influenza immunization 64
seasonal influenza 34
standard treatment 65–6
see also immunization
morbidity
bacterial (secondary) complications 38–9
excess deaths and consultations 1989–1999 **39**
influenza-like illness, weekly consultation rates **6**
RCGP data 38
severity and H3N2/H1N1 subtypes 12
statistics, websites 69
mortality
annual, UK 1
elderly persons 37
mouse, model of human infection 16
M_1 protein 5
M_2 protein 55
mucociliary escalator 16
mustelids
ferret, model of human infection 16
mink **22**, 24
Mycoplasma pneumoniae 64, 66, 67
myositis, children, clinical assessment 32

N-acetylneuraminic acid (Neu5Ac, NANA) 55
nasopharynx
ciliated epithelial cells
destruction by virus **16**
histopathology **17**

National Institute for Health and Clinical Excellence (NICE)
guidelines 61, 66
websites 69
Netherlands, cross-species transmission 26
neuraminidase 4–5
antigenic variability 9–10
N1, N2 antigens (pigs and humans) 21, **22**
N1–N9 (birds) **22**
N7, N8 antigens (horses) **22**
in non-human species 6, **22**
number (9) of NA proteins 11, 21–2
neuraminidase inhibitors 55–9
chemoprophylaxis 60
efficacy 57
structure and characteristics 57
treatment of community-acquired influenza 57–8
nomenclature 5
nucleocapsid protein 3, 4

oseltamivir 56–7
dosage **58**
prophylaxis 59–61, **60**
structure and characteristics 57
treatment of community-acquired influenza, NICE guidelines 58, 61, **66**

pandemics
dependency on genetic reassortment 11
endmatter 10–11
future, dependency on H5N1 mutations 22
pathogenesis 15–19, 38
clearance of virus 18–19
establishment of infection 15–16
interferon 17
local host factors 17–18
serum antibody 18
PB2 gene 26
perception of immunization 51–2
pigs *see* swine influenza
pneumonia 32–3, 66–7
clinical assessment 32–3
X-ray presentation 33
porcine respiratory tract, 'mixing' vessel 24
poutry infections *see* avian (type A) influenza
pregnancy, influenza in 34
primary infection, immunological memory 18
prophylaxis, with antiviral drugs 59–61

RCGP morbidity statistics 38
website 69
Relenza *see* zanamivir
residential care homes 67
resistance to infection 12–13
respiratory syncytial virus (RSV) 64, 67
respiratory tract epithelial cells
destruction by virus, animal models **16**
establishment of influenza virus **47**
specificity of receptors in avians and humans 25
Reye's syndrome, children, clinical assessment 32
rimantadine 55–6
prophylaxis 59–61
risk groups offered influenza immunization 43–4, **45**, **64**
chronic heart disease 64
chronic renal disease 64
chronic respiratory disease including asthma 64
diabetes 64
immunocompromised patients 37–41, 64
risk groups offered influenza prophylaxis 59
RNA, in virus structure 4–5
Russian flu (H1N1 subtype) epidemic 11

seals **22**, 24
serum antibody 18
sialic acid analogues (neuraminidase inhibitors) 55–9
smoking, bacterial complications 40
Spanish (swine) influenza pandemics 1, 10, 22
Staphylococcus aureus infection 37–8
appearance at postmortem of lung **38**
steroids, immunocompromised patients **64**
Streptococcus pneumoniae infection 37
structure
antiviral drugs 57
influenza virus particle 3, **4**
RNA of virus 4–5
swine (type A) influenza
clinical disease 27
cross-species transmission 22, 23
human/pig cross-transmission 30

swine (type A) influenza – (*continued*)
endemic H1N1 and H3N2 strains 24
epidemiology 23–4
H1, H3, N1, N2 antigens 24
H1N1, two different lineages 24
and porcine respiratory tract 24
"Spanish" pandemics 1, 10, 23
Symmetrel *see* amantadine

Tamiflu *see* oseltamivir
Thailand
cases and deaths 2003–2006 **30**, 35
tigers and leopards, cross-transmission 22, 27
trachea, ciliated epithelial cells, destruction by virus **16**
transcriptase complex 4
transmission
cross-species *v* 11, 22, 29–30
in humans 15
Turkey, avian influenza cross-transmission 23

vaccines *see* immunization
variability 1, 5
Vietnam 34
virulence factors 12, **26**
avian (type A) influenza 12, 24–5, **26**
influenza A virus 12
mutations of HA affecting cleavage 24–5

waders/wildfowl, adaptation to type A influenza viruses 21, 23
websites 69–70
whales **22**, 24, **28**
workplaces, complications of influenza 67
World Health Organization (WHO), website 70

zanamivir 56–7
dosage **58**
inhaled administration 59
prophylaxis 59–61, **60**
structure and characteristics 57
treatment of community-acquired influenza, NICE guidelines 58, **66**